A VICTORIAN GUIDE
TO
HEALTHY LIVING

A VICTORIAN GUIDE TO
HEALTHY LIVING

Thomas Allinson

Edited by Anna Selby

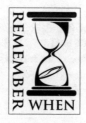

First published in Great Britain in 2009 by
REMEMBER WHEN
an imprint of
Pen & Sword Books Ltd
47 Church Street
Barnsley
South Yorkshire
S70 2AS

ISBN 978 1 84468 076 4

Printed and bound in the UK
by MPG Books

Pen & Sword Books Ltd incorporates the imprints of
Pen & Sword Aviation, Pen & Sword Maritime, Pen & Sword Military,
Wharncliffe Local History, Pen & Sword Select, Pen & Sword Military Classics,
Leo Cooper, Remember When, Seaforth Publishing and Frontline Publishing

For a complete list of Pen & Sword titles please contact
PEN & SWORD BOOKS LIMITED
47 Church Street, Barnsley, South Yorkshire, S70 2AS, England
E-mail: enquiries@pen-and-sword.co.uk
Website: www.pen-and-sword.co.uk

CONTENTS

INTRODUCTION

'YOU ARE what you eat' was an idea that came to prominence in the 1960s and if at first it was thought of as a bit cranky, it soon took hold of the popular imagination – to the extent that nowadays we have 'health gurus' examining the fridges, cupboards, bins (and even more intimate waste) of the hapless public. In fact, the phrase – or something very like it, 'A man is what he eats' – was first uttered by one Dr Thomas Richard Allinson who would have been over 100 had he survived to the decade it was aired the second time around.

To say that Allinson was a man before his time is putting it very mildly, though contrary to popular belief, the Nineteenth Century was an era when many new ideas and ways of living were tried on for size. He was not, for instance, the only advocate of vegetarianism. George Bernard Shaw, H. G. Wells and Charles Darwin were, too, and in the United States, a fellow doctor and vegetarian, John Harvey Kellogg, proposed a healthy way of life based on diet and exercise and became the inventor of the corn flake. It was at best though, regarded at the time as a somewhat eccentric way of life.

Allinson combined his role as doctor with that of a popular newspaper columnist and from 1885 wrote a column in *The Weekly Times and Echo*. He wrote books and gave lectures and achieved a huge following for his advice on 'hygienic medicine'– healthy food, regular exercise and fresh air – as a cure for most ills. This may seem like stating the obvious nowadays – but it was certainly not the view at a time when filth and squalor were the norm in Victorian cities. Industrial smoke and waste meant air pollution was rife. Food itself was often adulterated with chemicals and even poisons. The nation's health was appalling with 43 the average life expectancy and almost half of all babies and children dying before they reached their fifth birthday. Much of this, Allinson believed, could be traced back to the poor diet and conditions most people suffered.

His conclusion was 'hygienic medicine', a way of life that was regarded as radical at the time, even if today we take most of it for granted. His premises included that a healthy diet (lots of wholemeal bread, fruit and vegetables) resulted in a healthy life; everyone should take plenty of exercise; obesity was the result of overeating; tobacco was a cause of cancer (most doctors said it was good for you); and that the medicines of the day, largely based on mercury, opiates and arsenic, did more harm than good. Extraordinary as it seems today, these views were regarded at best as eccentric, at worst dangerous.

Championing diet and exercise as more effective cures than medicine was bad enough. But perhaps it was his belief that consulting a doctor was likely to do you more harm than good that brought him into the greatest conflict with his peers. Eventually accused of 'infamous professional conduct' he was struck off the Medical Register in 1892. But then he did accuse most doctors of 'being in the ranks of professional poisoners'.

He was to find himself in trouble with the law, too, and was prosecuted under the Obscene Prints Act for selling obscene literature. This was his 1901 pamphlet *A Book for Married Women* which championed women's rights, particularly the right of a woman to choose the size of her family and practise birth control. 'Women have rights as well as men, and to force a woman to have more children than her constitution will bear, or it is her desire to have, is an act of cruelty that no upright man would sanction.' The magistrate pronounced that it 'contained as much filth as could be compressed into a given space' and fined him £250.

Of course, not all of Allinson's views would be regarded favourably today. He was, for instance, a vigorous opponent of vaccination against smallpox. But no one can doubt the energy and conviction with which he championed a healthy diet or women's rights – ideas we now take for granted. However, Allinson is remembered less for his ground-breaking ideas than for the product that still bears his name today – wholemeal bread.

As part of his campaign for improving the nation's diet, in 1892 he bought a flour mill in Bethnal Green where he produced stone ground, wholemeal flour, campaigning against the white flour and bread that was so popular in Victorian England. White bread was widely believed to be the healthiest option at the time and wholemeal flour containing bran was thought to be bad for the digestive process. Chemicals were often added to the white bread to make it whiter still and the mills that produced it were far from clean. Allinson believed the grain should be stone ground and nothing – including the bran – should be discarded. He went on to found The Natural Food Company selling healthy foods. During the First World War, the value of whole grain bread was recognised and Allinson was offered the right to re-register as a doctor. He refused. His bread is still in the shops today.

Cold baths and three-hour walks in the rain may not be greeted too enthusiastically today but many of Allinson's ideas are now recognised as the foundation of health. So raise a glass – or should that be a cup of thin cocoa – to Dr Thomas Richard Allinson, pioneer of holistic medicine, champion of women's rights and founder of a flour empire.

Perhaps the best place to start to understand the man is in his essay entitled:

THE WAY I LIVE MY LIFE

I am an Englishman, born and bred in Lancashire, I studied and took my degree in Edinburgh, and came to London in 1880. I was born on March 29, 1858, and was married in 1888; my height is about 5ft 9in and my weight is about 9st 3lbs. I have been lighter in weight, but never much heavier.

I am of fair complexion, have a sandy beard, and a good head of hair, brushed back over my head, but not parted. I am full in the face, and my cheeks are ruddy; when walking I stoop a little from writing so much. My health is phenomenally good, but that is because I take care of it and live by rule. My spirits are always cheerful, and I have enough energy in me for two or three people.

I have not eaten any fish, flesh, or fowl since February 1882, as I find I can do my work much better without these things. When I first started life for myself, I had only my earnings to fall back on, and I found a non-flesh diet allowed me to make most of what little I had and what I earned; now I find such a diet allows me to make most out of my powers, and so I keep to it.

I am an abstainer from all alcoholic drinks. I find I cannot do mental work and drink any kind of alcoholic liquors. I want to make people teetotallers from my own standpoint. Let me feed people on brown bread, grain foods, vegetables and plenty of fruit, and I will make the people sober without a single temperance lecture, and without an Act of Parliament. If people will live properly, they will neither have a desire for strong liquor, nor will they take it.

As for tobacco, I do not use it. I gave it up in 1880 and from then until now I have only smoked once, then it made my mouth hot, parched my throat, and made me feel so queer about the head, that I have not touched it since.

Tea and coffee I have practically given up since 1886. I found they made me nervous, fidgety, anxious, low spirited, and took away some of my energy. Tea made me tremble, gave me brilliant but false ideas, and confused both speech and writing; coffee gave me wind and colic and took my memory away for four hours, so I have given both up. Salt, pepper, mustard, spices, condiments, pickles, and sauces I rarely use, as they are in some degree injurious and I have no craving for them.

I rise between 7 and 8am as a rule, and wash. While still wet, I dry my face, ears and neck, and then give my body a vigorous rubbing with the towel, and get it into a glow. My head gets washed only every three weeks, as I find too much soap causes scurf in the head, bleaches the hair, and makes it brittle. Occasionally I go in for a little mild exercise before dressing, such as throwing my arms about, or stooping in various ways to exercise the muscles. When dressed, I go out for half-an-hour's walk before breakfast, no matter how cold, wet or foggy.

My meals are three a day, about 9am, 3pm and 9pm. Breakfast consists of six ounces of brown bread, two apples, oranges or other fruit, and a cup of cocoa. I eat my food slowly, chew it well and eat bread and fruit together. At the end of my meal, I drink my cocoa, which is then nearly cool. I use Cadbury's cocoa, put half a teaspoonful in the cup, pour hot water over it, add one lump of white sugar and a tablespoonful of milk. Made thus it does not lead to biliousness nor does it repeat.

My dinner at 3pm varies a little. When I am using my brain more than usual I dine on bread and fruit. Two or three days a week I have a plain cooked diner, composed of a vegetable soup, milk pudding or stewed fruit. Tea, at 9pm, is a repetition of breakfast, for a change I may have beetroot, celery or boiled or fried onions.

On this simple diet, which will not cost a shilling a day, I work fourteen hours out of the twenty-four, am bright and merry at the end of the day, and have uninterrupted good health.

I walk from eight to twelve miles every day. Often on Sunday I manage to get in sixteen miles' walking. The weather never prevents me going out. I rarely wear an overcoat, except when it is wet or if I am travelling. At night I do not always wear my hat when walking, but let the cold air strengthen my scalp and keep my hair from falling off. Fresh air I try to get everywhere; in my bedroom and sitting-room the windows are always open three or four inches night and day, and in all weathers.

I go to bed as soon after midnight as I can, and just before jumping into bed I pull up the blinds. By this means I awake earlier and more fully; the light acts as a stimulant, and makes me feel cheerful. I never exclude the sun from my rooms.

My boots are broad at the toes, not tight fitting, the heels are low, and the soles fairly thick. I do not wear flannels, and only such clothes as protect the body from undue cold. The tall hat I abominate, but yet wear when making professional calls.

Now that I have given my readers an idea of how I live and why I do so, I hope they will take hints, and make themselves happier and healthier in consequence by my example.

T R Allinson

PART ONE: FOOD

Chapter I

THE STAFF OF LIFE

THE ALLINSON name lives on today in his bread and, as bread was the very cornerstone of his hygienic medicine, it seems a good place to start. His first collection of essays includes one entitled simply *Brown Bread*:

'In my lectures on Health I always advise my hearers to eat brown bread. Now what do I mean by brown bread and why do I recommend its use? By brown bread I mean wheatmeal or wholemeal bread, that is, the entire wheaten grain finely ground and made into bread by any of the known ways, with nothing left out, nor must it be made with chemicals. The reasons why we should use the entire grain are many. Wheat is a seed consisting of an outer covering, commonly called bran, and a starchy kernel from which white flour is made. The bran consists of innutritious ligneous or woody fibres, and also of most of the mineral matter of the wheat, such as the phosphates, iron &c. Just beneath the outer coat is a layer of cells containing much of the nitrogen in the grain and the great part of this, together with the mineral matter, is lost when we throw away the bran. The result is that by using white bread we get a food which is deficient in mineral matter, the flesh-forming material is in wrong proportions and we are not properly nourished. In consequence, our teeth decay early, our children often suffer from rickets, and we are not satisfied with our food. Mothers who are suckling their children should always eat brown bread, as it helps to form teeth and bones for the child. Rickets arise from a want of lime salts in the blood, and can only be cured by means of brown bread or oatmeal. Giving phosphate of lime alone will not cure. Milk used to be considered a type of perfect food; and so it is for young animals. The type of a perfect solid food for a grown up man is wheat. It contains vegetable nitrogen, for building up muscles; starch for giving heat and force; mineral salts, for bones, teeth &c and a certain amount of innutritious matter which causes a daily action of the bowels. Brown bread and water contain everything necessary for a hard working life. Persons who eat white bread often suffer from an inward craving or sinking; to cure this, recourse is often had to beer, wine or spirits, which lulls the craving for a time. If they ate brown bread they would not suffer from this and we should have a more sober nation.

'Now, leaving aside the chemical nature of the bran, we come to another point, its use mechanically. The innutritious bran has two very important uses. First, it separates the particles of food and allows the gastric and various intestinal juices to penetrate, and so thoroughly to dissolve all the possible nutriment from the food we eat; and next, by its bulk it helps to fill the stomach, and keeps us from eating too much. It also aids in filling up the small intestines, and stimulates the involuntary muscles of the bowels, thus causing daily laxation. One great curse of this country is constipation which is caused in a great measure by white bread. From constipation arises back-ache, piles, varicocele, varicose veins and ulcers &c; while from the bile and other intestinal excretions not being daily got rid of, we get headache, irritability, dullness, miserable feelings &c... .

'Separating the bran from the flour may be said to have come into fashion at the beginning of the century and as a consequence, pill factories arose, and are now almost a necessary part of the State. Would you banish the pill box from your private cupboard? Then you must drive white bread from your table. All who are naturally costive should use brown bread. I have cured thousands of long-standing cases of constipation simply by its use. Growing children should always eat it, as it forms bones for them, and prevents straining at stool, which sometimes causes falling of the bowel. Adults should use it, as by causing laxation it will leave their heads clearer for their business. Old persons should always use it, as straining of stool in the old may give rise to a stroke of apoplexy.'

Allinson follows this with an essay on *Bread and Bread Making* in which he explains what makes bread wholemeal – as he produced in his own mill:

'I am sorry to say it, but many of the samples of bread sent to me have been simply a mixture of bran and white flour. In some cases mixtures of pollards, seconds and flour. To get a perfect bread five things are necessary:

1st Your materials must be of the best kind.
2nd These must be finely ground.
3rd Nothing must be taken away.
4th Nothing injurious must be added.
And 5th The bread should be well baked.

'I: Only the best materials must be used or the bread will be inferior in flavour and in nourishing qualities. The stuff called wholemeal used by some bakers is nothing but damaged and inferior flour. In France and Germany, bad wheat gives rise to a very distressing condition, known as ergotism, from the ergot of rye being in the flour; whilst in Italy a disease known as pellagra is brought on by eating diseased Indian corn. A mixture of foreign and English wheats gives a better bread, than if either is used separately.

'II: It must be finely ground. What disgusts many people with wholemeal bread is its coarseness and roughness. Some bread one sees looks as if the wheat had simply been crushed and made into loaves. This is wrong. If the wheat is finely ground, we digest it quicker, get more nutriment from it and our intestines are not irritated by big pieces of bran. Coarse bread causes too loose a condition of the bowels, and so the food is carried off before we get all the nutrient matter from it.

'III: Nothing must be removed. There are granulated, decorticated and other breads in the market. In all of these a portion of the bran has been removed. This is wrong for the bran has beneficial uses. In the first place, the bran contains mineral matter useful in forming bone and teeth and for the blood; next, the particles of bran give bulk to the food, fill up the intestines, allow the intestinal juices to penetrate into and around the food; and lastly, they also act as a stimulant to the intestinal muscles, and so cause daily action of the bowels. When the entire bran is removed some of the flesh-forming part of the wheaten grain is lost and nearly all the mineral matter.

'IV: Nothing must be added. An unleavened and aerated bread would be the best if of the entire meal, but I know of none. The next simplest process is to use yeast as a raiser. I object to the various chemical raisers as they may contain impurities, and even if pure do not properly unite, and our teeth and internal organs are injured by the chemicals employed. The ordinary raisers used are baking powders composed of bicarbonate of soda, tartaric acid and powdered rice. This raises bread nicely, but leaves in your loaf tartrate of soda, or even uncombined soda. This soda helps on rheumatism, gout, stone in bladder, kidneys and gall bladder, and produces other evils as well... . A more scientific mixture is hydrochloric or muriatic acid and bicarbonate of soda. The union of these is supposed to leave only common salt in the bread after raising it. In practice there is always an excess of either acid or soda. The latter gives rise to the evils mentioned above and the former is in itself a poison and frequently contains arsenic... .

'V: Bread should be well baked. A well-baked loaf keeps sweet longer, and is easier of digestion than one half baked. It need not be made light and spongy. There is really no objection to a solid hard loaf except that time is required to chew it... .

'To get pure wheatmeal, the best plan is to have a wheat mill and grind the wheat yourself. Such a mill can be obtained from any large ironmonger. By means of it you are independent of the miller. Good wholemeal bread is made thus: - Put in a bread mug about seven pounds of wholemeal flour. Make a hole in the centre of the flour, and into this pour a quart of warm water, in which half an ounce of German yeast has been dissolved. Gradually stir flour and yeast together until well mixed into a dough, and allow to ferment an hour before the fire. Then add a little more water and a little salt, one or two tablespoonfuls to taste. Knead well again, let it stand for another hour in front of the fire, then fill your bread tins from this, and bake about an hour. A little experience and a few trials will soon make perfect.'

In his third collection of essays, Allinson includes wholemeal bread as the principal item in one entitled *Perfect Foods*, where he explains just why he believes it is so well suited to man's metabolism and reveals himself – yet again long before his time – as a champion of whole foods in all forms (not to mention, militant in his fight against constipation):

'Every animal in its natural state has one or more foods on which it lives, and these he eats in a natural condition. Thus, the lion eats the flesh and smaller bones of the animals it kills. In the Dublin Zoological Gardens they rear lions more successfully than anywhere else because they feed them on goats. The lion can, to a certain extent, eat the bones as well as the flesh of these animals, and so is perfectly nourished. The cow eats grass and from it gets all she wants for her blood, bones, muscles, also fat to keep her warm. Fowls eat entire grains. Even the young chick absorbs some of the shell in which it was contained before being hatched. Uncivilised man eats all parts of the food on which he lives. It is only when individuals form communities, and a fashion in foods is set, that he departs from his natural condition. Nowadays there is scarcely a single article of food that is not emasculated or altered from the condition in which it is supplied by Nature. This custom of eating only parts of food is injurious and leads to disastrous results. The excess of one particular substance in our food means disease due to this excess; whilst deficiency of another part means loss of bodily function or impaired nutrition. There are also some substances in our food which are difficult to be got rid of, and set up disease, unless they carry with them their own dissolvers or solvents.

'Let us examine by the above fact the bread eaten by the ordinary Englishman. My readers are no doubt aware that I brand white bread as an imperfect, and, therefore, unwholesome article of food. Why do I do this? Because white bread is only a partial food. It is rich in starch, but very deficient in nitrogen, mineral matter and insoluble vegetable fibre. What would be the result if a person lived only on white bread and water? The first result would be obstinate constipation. This is because the bran is removed from the flour before white bread can be made from it. This bran is the natural laxative in our food. It cures constipation by simulating the bowels to act, and by being insoluble it fills up the intestines, gives bulk, and is thus the cause of daily action.

The next result would be that the man would lose strength. White flour does not contain much nitrogen, or muscle forming material. The man would consequently feel weak, have little energy, and be unfit for doing much work. Lastly, his bones and teeth would suffer as white flour is deficient in bone-forming material. It is said that dogs fed on white bread die from starvation in six weeks. Whether this is exactly true or not I cannot say; but I do know that the animal would suffer much in consequence. A dog fed on brown bread would be no worse for the experiment.

'Eat brown bread in its entirety. Grind the wheat as fine as ever you please, but do not have anything removed... . The other foods in common use must be taken as nearly as possible as they come from nature. Oats are best ground finely or coarsely, according to the purpose for which they are used. Do not buy prepared oats, nor those brands whose makers boast that they have removed a part that is not digestible. The insoluble part of food is necessary for the proper functions of nutrition and digestion. Barley, maize and other grains must, for the same reason, be taken as pure and perfect as we can get them... .

'The imperfect foods made from wheat are white flour and its preparations, also macaroni, semolina, and gluten bread. Macaroni and semolina are better foods than white flour, because, being richer in nitrogen, they contain more flesh formers, but being deprived of bran they are constipating. For this reason I always advise macaroni to be eaten with prunes or a green vegetable. Maize meal is eaten in Italy and is called polenta. Hominy, samp and cornflour are made from maize, but are only parts of the grain; their use should be restricted. Fruits are good, wholesome, and blood-purifying foods; generally speaking the skins should be eaten, as in the skin lies much mineral matter, also insoluble particles which prevent constipation. Thus the rinds or skins of apples, pears, peaches, plums, apricots, grapes, cherries, gooseberries and currants should be eaten. The skins of lemons, oranges, pomegranates and bananas must be rejected, as these do not form part of the fruit, but only a covering for it.

'Cooked vegetables we should also eat as much as possible in their entirety. Thus the leaves of cabbages and cauliflowers should be eaten, likewise the skins of carrots, turnips and even potatoes. Wash them clean and you have nothing to fear. Peel potatoes, cook and eat them, and you find them constipating. Wash your potatoes, roast them and then eat the browned skin, and you will find them more satisfying than peeled ones and not so constipating.

'When we consider animal products, we find that eggs and milk are fairly good foods, meant rather for the growing calf or chick than man. We can use them in moderation with benefit. Milk we find subjected to many processes, and various products got from it, as cream, butter and cheese. When we separate these things from the milk and eat them, we get an unbalanced dietary. Cream is only so much grease or fat, and when taken into the system as a food it cannot all be used up. Some find that it produces acidity of the stomach, in others its presence causes pimples, boils and skin eruptions and if its use is long continued it helps to cause stoutness, or form fatty and sebaceous tumours and gall stones. What has been said of cream is also applicable to butter. The habit of eating butter with bread is purely one of custom; there is no reason for it in nature or on physiological grounds. When one eats good wholemeal bread there is no necessity for butter at all. If much butter is used on bread, then it causes some of the complaints I name above. Cheese contains most of the fat and curd of milk, with added salt. It is very indigestible food, as it is so close grained. It contains excess of nitrogen and if much of it is eaten disposes to gravelly urine, to stone in bladder, kidneys or gall bladder or even gout and rheumatism. Eaten in small quantity and well masticated it will not do much harm.

'When we come to consider flesh as food, we find that as an article of diet it is very imperfect. It consists chiefly of fat and nitrogen, and these not in the proportion of a food proper for man. Flesh contains very little lime salts for the bones. Thus when persons dine on white bread, meat and peeled potatoes, with cornflour and say apple rings, they make a most unsatisfactory meal. It is constipating, deficient in laxative and saline matter and must upset the system. Human beings have no right to eat flesh, and those who value their health will not do so.

'Sugar is another imperfect food, it being a sweet extract of the sugar cane. It is looked upon almost as a necessity. Its use, especially in those who live indoors, leads to want of energy, acidity, flatulence, heartburn, pimples, blotches, boils and headaches. It also helps on eczema, boils, carbuncles, fatty and sebaceous tumours, stoutness and the other complaints mentioned under the results due to cream.

'**MORAL** – Eat all foods as nearly as possible as Nature provides them, avoid the artificial ones, and then you will be well, happy, energetic and long lived.'

Chapter 2

VEGETARIANISM

A S MUST be clear from the previous chapter, Allinson was no carnivore. In fact, he was a vegetarian from his twenties until the end of his life and this was principally based on his belief that the human body was simply not designed to eat meat – and if it did, trouble would surely follow. This was, of course, at the time regarded as eccentric at best, and most medical men believed it to be positively dangerous, recommending concoctions such as beef tea (see page 40) for invalids who couldn't eat solid food but could still thus get the benefits of meat. Allinson, on the contrary, believed that meat caused nothing but problems and fruit and vegetables – again, at the time regarded as foods to eat with caution and in minimal quantities – were far more beneficial. He argues his case in his essay, *The Truth about Vegetarianism*:

'The question of diet is one that must attract the attention of every thinking person at some time or other of his life, and as there are certain people who will not take steps of any kind until they are satisfied everything is safe, so there are others who rush in blindly where angels fear to tread. For both these classes and for the public generally I write upon this subject from a purely rational view. We may define a vegetarian as one who does not kill an animal for food, nor will he cause animals to be killed for food, but he may eat animal products, such as eggs, milk, butter, cheese and honey. A vegetarian thus makes an artificial distinction of foods. He eats eggs which may contain potent life and he drinks milk meant for a young calf, but he will not eat the producers of these foods. Life is no criterion to go by, for the vegetarian who eats a bit of cabbage may destroy hundreds of lives on that cabbage and when he drinks any country water, he may swallow an aquatic multitude. The difference between animals and plants is purely an arbitrary one, for where plant life ends and animal life begins is unknown to the scientist. Many plants are higher in intelligence than some animals, and though I myself firmly believe that the primitive diet of man was fruit and grain, yet there are some persons who would like to argue that man has really sprung from flesh-eating ancestors.

'Now, amongst all these conflicting arguments to whom or to what fact shall we appeal? To facts; on facts only can we place any reliance. Now what do facts prove as regards this question? Facts show that a man can live healthily and be strong on a diet into which flesh does not enter. First, with regard to strength, this country contain hundreds of hard working men who never eat any fish, flesh, or fowl, from year's end to year's end. Blacksmiths, porters, miners, carpenters, fishermen, puddlers, agricultural labourers &c are found in the ranks of the Vegetarian Society; whilst its roll contains the names of many men known to intellectual fame. Thus strength of body and mind are compatible with a non-flesh diet.

'Now with regard to health. My own experience and researches show me that a properly selected non-flesh diet is the best for health. I have inquired into the subject and I find that the non-flesh eater suffers from less illness than the mixed feeder. Again, experience has shewn me that in many severe cases of stomach, liver and kidney disease, it was only by such a non-flesh diet that I could do any good. In the majority of cases the result has been most satisfactory, and many persons are now hale and well who before were partially disabled. No one who adopts a non-flesh diet must expect to lose all his ailments by this simple diet alone. Many vegetarians come to consult me, but only a small proportion from their ranks as compared with those who are meat eaters... . The chief evils that the vegetarian escapes are constipation, piles and varicose veins. Indigestion, stomach and liver complaints do not trouble him much as a rule, whilst kidney complaints are uncommon. In other words, he escapes most of the plethoric diseases, or complaints due to overfeeding. His wounds and bruises usually heal quicker than those of a mixed feeder... .

'Again, what is flesh but grains and vegetables? To the philosophic inquirer all flesh is only grass under another form or name, whilst experience shows him that a non-flesh eater can live and work at less cost than a mixed feeder, and has better health. When a person asks me if it is safe to be a non-flesh eater, I answer it is, only he must be a rational one and live on scientific lines. He must take cereals in place of flesh and must eat peas, beans or lentils daily in small quantities, or in average quantities every other day. He must also eat fruits and vegetables freely. But beware of vegetarianism as a religion or a fad. In these cases it is injurious and liable to lead one astray but as a rational way of living there is none better.'

In 1889, in his second collection of essays, Allinson wrote of his own experiences as a vegetarian:

'More than seven-and-a-half years have now passed since I ate any fish, flesh or fowl and I think my experience may be of use in helping my readers on to health. I was not ill, nor in low condition when I began my present diet and have kept in good health ever since. The low, miserable feelings I used to suffer from have left me, and I find that my diet gives me more energy and more vitality in body and mind. I find I can do a great deal more mental work on it than on a mixed diet, and as for bodily powers, I have walked twenty-four miles in the day besides doing my ordinary work. So far it has suited me well.

'My first enquiry was into the condition of so-called vegetarians, that is persons who abstain from fish, flesh and fowl, but who take butter, eggs, milk and cheese in moderation. I find they are a clear and clean-skinned set of people whose faces vary in colour from a deep red to pale, like ordinary mortals. Their mental condition is good, they are all-round thinkers, and consequently are as a rule an intelligent set. Most of the vegetarians I know earn their living with their brains; but I know vegetarian miners, sailors, policemen, ironworkers, and labourers and one of my converts is working at a gasworks and lifting twenty-one tons of stuff a day. Students and literary men, or those whose occupation is sedentary (as clerks), gain more benefit from the adoption of a non-flesh diet. With regard to size of families, I find they have the average number. They also rear more children than the average mixed feeder. With regard to longevity, they are more likely to live longer than the ordinary meat feeder. The health of the vegetarian is better than that of the meat eater, and there are good reasons for this. The vegetarian is not content with abstaining from eating meat; the rule is for him not to smoke and not to take stimulants. He also believes in fresh air, regular exercise and bathing. He does not generally believe in vaccination, nor does he poison himself with drugs when ill, but relies on Nature and hygiene. If a person becomes a vegetarian only, then I hold him less in my esteem than another person who eats meat in moderation and obeys all the hygienic rules... .

'The temper of the vegetarian is good as a rule, and he takes a more cheerful view of life than his meat-eating friend. Excessive stoutness is a disease almost unknown among vegetarians; some are very thin but that will often be found to be due to their previous history or trying to live on uncooked grain, or something else to which they are unsuited. I have studied the vegetarian mode of living from a doctor's standpoint and my conclusions are that, if intelligently carried out, it is the best diet a man can adopt.'

In a later essay entitled *New Year Resolutions* he encourages his readers to give it a try, even in a small and gradual way:

'Many, thinking that flesh meat is necessary for life, spend their hard-earned money on it, get little nourishment in proportion to the money laid out, and so cannot compete in the struggle for existence with those who do not use it as food. Those who do not know this fact may leave off butcher's meat one day a week, and eat instead some well-boiled macaroni, or have some haricot beans boiled with onion, and eaten with vegetables; or make a vegetable pie of potatoes, onion and boiled haricot beans, soaked sago, sage, thyme or marjoram, a little butter, pepper and salt. When they find they can live one day without meat, they may next try doing without it two days a week and so on until they leave it off altogether; it will repay them in health and wealth to do so.'

Chapter 3

WHAT TO EAT

DURING the Nineteenth Century, fruit was regarded with caution. It was widely believed eating it could lead to stomach upsets or worse and was generally thought to be particularly dangerous when eaten raw. As a result, when it did form part of the diet, it was usually in the shape of a cooked pudding or as a preserve. Allinson was a great believer in eating as much of it as possible, in its natural state – unlike most doctors of the day. Indeed, he offered it in his essay *Fruit* as a more palatable alternative to most of his colleagues and their cures:

'The majority of people are fond of fruit and would eat freely of it were it not for the fact that they are afraid of ill results. Children are proverbially fond of fruit, and they will eat it in any stage from unripeness to decay. This craving for fruit is a natural one and should be satisfied. Where people live in a fair average way they may eat it freely and experience no ill results. The secret of fruit eating is that one should make a meal of it instead of finishing up a meal with it. After one has had meat and pudding to repletion, perhaps washed down with strong liquors, then he may eat a strawberry or two, and feel upset; the cause is the heavy food, not the light fruit. Here is a pleasant way of taking fruit and getting the full benefit of it: make a meal of dry brown bread and fruit, it may be breakfast, lunch or tea. Any of these meals may consist of dry brown bread with cherries, strawberries, gooseberries, plums or whatever is in season. The reason I ask persons to eat dry bread with it is to bring out the full flavour of the fruit. If butter is on the bread, then the salt in the butter or the flavour of the butter itself spoils that of the fruit. When a meal like this is made, no fluids are required. To the person weary of ordinary food I cannot recommend a more pleasant change. Try this plan with children on Saturdays or half-holidays when they are in the way at home. Buy them some good ripe fruit, give them some brown bread with a bottle of milk and water, and send them off to the park, common or other place where they can play. The fruit and bread is for their food. Older children may make use of the same hint for picnics and take a goodly supply of fruit with them.

'Fruit contains the same nourishment as other foods, only not in so concentrated a form. Fruit consists chiefly of water, containing from 70 to 90 per cent, a fair proportion of sugar, a little nitrogenous material, vegetable acids and salts and insoluble matter. Fruit may be said to be a perfect food for a state of indolence. It contains enough nourishment to keep a person in health if he is not doing much; and as it consists of so large a percentage of water, thirst is not experienced by those who eat freely of it. Fruit is invaluable to the system in hot weather, as it supplies it with fluid, and not containing any fat or other very heating material, the body itself does not generate so much heat and is therefore cooler.

'The vegetable acids of fruits are useful for making lime and soda salts soluble, which can then be thrown out of the system, and so getting rid of gall stones, stone in the bladder or kidneys, or other diseases due to the presence of these salts in the blood. The vegetable salts that fruits contain are also necessary to the system, which they supply with mineral water in a form it can use, and were fruits always used there would be no such thing as scurvy and scorbutic complaints. Fruits are good in constipation. The skins of fruit such as of the apple, pear, plum, cherry, gooseberry, and grape should always be eaten, as these contain the vegetable salts, and being insoluble themselves, they help to cause daily action of the bowels; fruit should not be eaten in the evening. An early tea is the last meal at which it should be taken. In France and Germany there is the 'grape cure' for many diseases, and indeed it is invaluable in many complaints. To carry it out properly one should live in the country the whole time while undergoing it and eat freely of ripe fruit. In Germany a person begins with eating a pound or two of grapes with bread and increases the quantity of grapes until he can eat half a dozen or more pounds during the day. Of course very little bread is eaten as more grapes are taken. This is a famous cure for obesity and diseases due to high living. In Germany during the cherry season the druggists' takings are said to be only half the usual amount.

'My readers now, I hope, will see the value of fruit as a food and as a corrective of a disordered condition of the system, and they should not let a day pass without taking fruit with at least one meal.'

Allinson, in his third collection of essays, elaborates on the theme of fruit as an alternative to the prescribed medicines of the day:

'If we will only eat a fair amount of fresh fruit daily, we shall have little need to trouble the doctor or the druggist. Many people look at it and desire to eat it, but ignorance and fear say "Do not touch it". Diarrhoea, with upset of the stomach bowels, is supposed to follow the eating of it. This is a mistake. Ripe raw fruit is one of the best correctives and curative agents we have. Where it is made part of the dietary no harm can or does result but immense beneficial changes occur and the body is often freed from disease. Persons can live on fruit alone but it is not wise to do so; being chiefly composed of water, a large quantity would have to be eaten and too much energy would be wasted in its absorption and digestion. But when eaten with grain foods, it forms an ideal diet... .

'From an aesthetic aspect, a table set with good wholesome brown bread, and a tempting array of ripe fruits is surely more pleasing than one laid out with carcases of dead animals, sodden vegetables and sloppy messes called puddings. From a gustatory or taste point of view the same must be said... . In fact, most of the cooked meat dishes are so many excuses for irritating our taste nerves by means of condiments. What a difference also from a rational point of view. A fruit and bread meal is eaten with relish; the mind is free to occupy itself, whilst the associations of fruit lead one to pleasant ideas. One rises from such a meal satisfied without being heavy and knowing that he has not laden the stomach with food that will burden it, and tax the other organs to get rid of it.

'How and when should we eat fruits? Fruits are best eaten ripe, raw and at the first two meals. Raw fruit at night is apt to lie heavily, and cause dreams and a nasty taste in the mouth; five hours should always be allowed before one goes to bed after a fruit meal, unless the fruit is stewed, then three hours must pass... . About a pound of fruit is a fair daily quantity. Say, half a pound both at breakfast and tea time.

Those who will live on bread and fruit only may eat another half-pound at dinner… . Give children plenty of fruit; money spent on it will be saved from doctors' bills.'

The Tomato

The tomato, though often regarded as a salad vegetable, is actually a fruit. It was introduced to Europe during the sixteenth century but was long regarded as dangerous. Even a hundred years later, it was thought to cause gout and cancer. And during the Victorian period, no less an authority than Mrs Beeton thought tomatoes rather dangerous and likely to cause 'vertigo and vomiting'. Allinson, however, recommended them:

'The tomato belongs to the same class of plants as the potato and tobacco. The fruit of the tomato plant is in composition very like the apple. It contains a large quantity of water, a small percentage of sugar and of colouring matter and a medium amount of malic acid. As it comes in some time before apples are ripe it may well take their place for many purposes and as it contains less sugar than apples it can be eaten when the latter disagree.

'**Medicinal uses**: As a food it is invaluable in all kinds of calcareous disease, that is, in cases where lime, magnesia or other mineral salts are in excess in the body. For this reason it is invaluable in stone in the kidney, stone in the bladder, gall stones, gravel, and all thick conditions of the urine. Gout and rheumatism are also lessened by the use of tomatoes. Acidity of the stomach is decreased by their use, especially if they are used instead of butter as a means of helping down bread. Many find that they cause dreams if eaten late at night, so an early tea is the last meal at which they should be eaten. The daily allowance should not exceed a pound a day. Many persons do not like their taste at first, but soon get accustomed it and then find them delicious. Tomatoes are said to favour the development of cancer. I have tried to find an authority and the origin of this untrue rumour, but cannot discover either. The same was said of potatoes when first introduced. At one time tomatoes were thought to contain a poisonous acid called oxalic, but later analysis has shown that this is not the case… .

'**How to cook**: Tomatoes are best in their natural condition, and should be eaten with bread the same as an apple. This is the best way to eat them. They are very good also to eat with plain raw cucumber or with lettuce. A very nice salad is made from lettuce, one hard boiled egg, tomatoes, oil, vinegar, pepper and salt and those who like onions can make it more tasty by adding these to the salad. One large head of lettuce will need half a pound of tomatoes mixed with it. Tomato salad and brown bread make a good midday meal. Some use pepper and vinegar with tomatoes, but they are best eaten plain. Some also eat them with sugar, but I think any addition spoils them. Others again cut them in slices with onion, and add pepper, vinegar and olive oil to them and use as a relish to cold meat; I do not think they are so good this way. Tomatoes may be grilled, fried or stewed. A simple way of cooking them is to put them in a pie dish in the oven with a little water, butter, pepper and salt and let them bake. Then eat with other vegetables or having steamed some rice, put the baked tomatoes on the rice; pour the tomato juice over and serve as a savoury.'

Macaroni

Allinson was an early British advocate of pasta and the Mediterranean diet, as was evidenced in his praise of Macaroni – by which he means all pasta:

'Patients and correspondents occasionally ask why I recommend macaroni so much, seeing it is made from white flour. I will give now my reasons. Ordinary wheat contains about twelve per cent of nitrogen or twelve parts in a hundred or a little over two ounces to the pound, whilst wheat from which macaroni is made contains twenty per cent or twenty parts in a hundred or not quite four ounces to the pound. From this we learn the immense value of macaroni as a flesh-forming food; it also contains a large amount of starch, and a reasonable amount of bone-forming matter. Only a little of the bran is taken away in the milling.

'Here is the average composition of the wheat from which macaroni is made:

Nitrogen	20
Carbon	65
Mineral Matter	3
Water	12
	100

Compare this with lean meat:

Nitrogen	19
Carbon	4
Mineral Matter	5
Water	72
	100

'From this we see that whilst macaroni contains as much flesh-forming matter as meat, it also contains sixteen times as much heat and force-forming material as does flesh. Fat, of which lean meat contains four per cent, has two and a half times more force-producing matter than starch – that is if the fat is digested and absorbed.

'It is a fact that one pound of macaroni contains more nourishment than four pounds of butcher's meat. The macaroni is pure, wholesome, will keep and is not dear. The flesh is always more or less diseased, may contain parasites, tapeworms, or other creatures, will not keep and besides being an unwholesome food, is very dear for the little nourishment it contains.

'To make a perfect food of macaroni it must be eaten with fruit or with vegetables to take the place of the bran removed. If the poor and working classes would eat more macaroni and less meat they would be better in health, spirits and pocket and there would be less temptation for them to go to the public house. Buy the Italian macaroni either in coils, tubes or strips; the cost is from 3d to 8d a pound. It is a suitable food for the strong as well as for the weak. Being a close knit food it must be well cooked and chewed so that it may not lie heavy in the stomach.'

'**How to cook pasta**: Allinson was very keen on Italian pasta but not on the Italian way of cooking it. *Al dente* was not a term he would have comprehended and he served it as often as a sweet dish as a savoury one:

'The usual method is by putting it into boiling water for half an hour. Invalids may soak it in plain cold water overnight and then it will only require ten or 15 minutes cooking in the water in which it was soaked. When done it may be eaten with milk and stewed prunes, or other fruit, or it may be eaten plain with baked potatoes and any kind of vegetables; it is specially nice with fried onions, tomatoes or mushrooms. To make a savoury course of it, put the cooked macaroni into a pie dish, mix some wholemeal flour in the water in which it was cooked, an egg, chopped onion or parsley and a little pepper and salt; pour this over the macaroni and bake in the oven. When done eat with brown onion sauce and vegetables. If grated cheese is mixed with the batter or sprinkled on the top before it is baked we get macaroni cheese. A better way is to grate the cheese and sprinkle it on the macaroni on your plate. If the macaroni is put into a pie dish, then egg and milk beaten up together with spice and a little sugar poured over it and it is allowed to set in the oven, we have a macaroni pudding.

'Here is a tasty tea dish: boil macaroni, drain and put in a mould, stir some tapioca or sago in the water in which the macaroni was boiled and cook this until it thickens; then add salt, pepper and nutmeg to taste, pour this over the macaroni and let it cool. Then turn out on a dish and garnish with parsley. This makes a very good imitation of brawn and is very savoury; eat with bread and vegetables. Dozens of other macaroni dishes can be made by the skilful housewife. At Christmas, after being cooked, it can take the place of tripe that some people put in with their mince-meat. Working men can take it with them to work as it eats very well cold either as a pudding or savoury.'

Salads

Allinson was keen, too, on vegetables and advised eating salads as often as possible, though these could be made of cooked as well as raw vegetables:

'Salads can be eaten all the year round, but they will be found most acceptable in hot weather. They can be composed of any kind of vegetables or green stuff, either raw or cooked. I now write chiefly of those salads most suitable for summer use and will give their constituents. These dishes being usually made of vegetables and green stuff in an uncooked condition, contain all the nourishment of the plants in its natural state, and being raw they have in them the unchanged vegetable acids and their mineral matter is not boiled out of them. As they contain a large proportion of pure water, they help to prevent thirst; and, not being very nourishing, they supply bulk and prevent us from overfeeding in the hot weather. They are also appetising. We can thus tickle our palate with them and get our bread down instead of having recourse to cheese, pickles, salted or smoked foods. Salads may be eaten at any meal but lunch, dinner or tea are the usual meals at which they are taken. We can satisfy our hunger with salad and bread or it may take the place of a vegetable at dinner or form one of the ordinary courses of a meal.

'**Composition**: Summer salads are chiefly composed of lettuce and to this is added a large variety of other things. In making these dishes, we must take care to have all the greens thoroughly clean and dry. The lettuce must have all the damaged leaves removed and the sound ones carefully washed in fresh or salt water, leaf by leaf, so that no worms, caterpillars or sand are left in them. They are then allowed to drain, or are dried with a towel; after this, they are cut up finely and put into the salad bowl. Then a teaspoonful of vinegar and a tablespoonful of olive or salad oil are added, the whole mixed together with a wooden spoon and fork and your simple salad is ready. Those who like salt may add a little. To make the salad more savoury, wash and clean spring onions, cut them up fine and mix with the lettuce. A more complicated salad is to mix finely cut lettuce, onions, radish, mustard and cress, or watercress together. Some make a further addition to this of hard-boiled eggs, cut into slices and mixed with the greens. Taking lettuce as the foundation of the salad, you can add to it almost anything. Sorrel, or sour dock, as it is sometimes called, or wood sorrel, gives a pleasant acidity. Cucumber, tomatoes, beetroot, cold potatoes, etc can all be mixed up and made into salads. Lemon juice is added by some, instead of vinegar and is more wholesome. The elaborate salad dressings made with mustard, vinegar, oil, cream, sugar, salt and eggs beaten up are not to be recommended, as the addition of these things turns a simple salad into an indigestible compound.

'Cold vegetables make a pleasant salad for tea. Thus, cold sliced green beans, cold peas or cold cauliflower can be mixed with lettuce, oil, vinegar and salt and make a good relish at tea-time, which is not too heavy in the hot weather. In winter, potato salads are very useful. Cold boiled potatoes are cut into slice; sliced beetroot and cut fine onion are also added, a little watercress is put with these and then the oil and vinegar poured over and mixed. Lobster salads and such things are abominations that my readers will do well to avoid unless they want indigestion, diarrhoea etc. To put even fine cheese into a salad makes it too heavy, the only animal product that should go into a salad being hard-boiled egg.

'A not unpleasant salad is orange salad; it is composed of oranges peeled and pipped and mixed with boiled and sliced beetroot, it is a splendid help to get down dry brown bread... . Everyone may with great benefit eat two salad dinners a week in summer; that is, have only half a pound of brown bread and a dish of salad for dinner. Those who want a relish at tea time which will not lie heavily, nor heat their blood too much, nor keep them awake at night, cannot do better than have one of these dishes. Salads should be made only just before they are wanted and never eaten if more than twelve hours old. Salads are beneficial, as they help to prevent stones in the kidney, bladder or elsewhere and to dissolve them if formed; and they tend to make soluble the uric acid products that cause rheumatism and gout.'

Wholemeal Cookery

At a time when people made their own pastry, pies and sauces themselves, rather than buying foods that were ready made, Allinson extended his advice on eating wholemeal bread to using wholemeal flour wherever possible:

'Most of my readers have received great benefit from eating wholemeal bread instead of white, and they may all gain further good if they will use finely ground wholemeal flour in place of white for all cooking purposes. Those who are at all constipated, or who suffer from piles, varicose veins, varicocele, back pain etc, should never use white flour in cooking. Those who are inclined to stoutness should use wholemeal flour rather than white. Hygienists and health reformers should not permit white flour to enter their houses unless it is to make bill-stickers' paste or some like stuff. Mothers often bake white flour for their babies and give them this; they can bake wholemeal flour in the same way and give their children and then a perfect food is supplied to them. Toothless children must not be given any food but milk and water until they have cut at least two teeth.

'Every kind of cookery can be done with fine wholemeal flour. In making ordinary white sauce or vegetable sauce, this is how we make it: chop fine some onion or parsley; boil in a small quantity of water, stir in wholemeal flour and milk, add a little pepper and salt, thin with hot water, and you will have an excellent sauce to help down vegetables and potatoes. In making a brown sauce we put a little butter or olive oil in the frying pan, let it bubble and sputter, dredge in wholemeal flour, stir it round with a knife until browned, then add boiling water, pepper, salt, a little ketchup and you then have a nice brown sauce for many dishes. If we wish to make it very tasty, we fry a finely chopped onion first and add that to it. White sweet sauce is made from wholemeal flour, milk, sugar and a little cinnamon, cloves, lemon juice, vanilla or other flavourings. Yorkshire puddings, Norfolk dumplings, batter puddings and similar puddings can all be made with wholemeal flour and are more staying, nourishing and healthy and do not lie so heavily on the stomach as those made from white flour. Pancakes can be made from wholemeal flour just as well as from white flour.

'All kinds of pastry, pie crusts, under crusts &c are best made from this flour, but if much butter, lard, or dripping is used they will lie just as heavy, and cause heartburn just as much as those made with white flour. We have a substitute for pie crust that is very tasty and not at all harmful. We call it 'batter' and it can be used for savoury dishes as well as for sweet ones. Here are a few recipes for savoury dishes: fry some potatoes, then some onions, put them in layers in a pie dish; next make a batter of wholemeal flour, one or two eggs, milk and a little pepper with salt, pour over the fried vegetables as they lie in the dish, bake in the oven from half an hour to an hour, until in fact, the batter has formed a crust; eat with the usual vegetables. Or chop fine cold vegetables of any kind, fry onions and put with the vegetables, put in a pie dish, pour some of the batter over them and bake. All kinds of scraps can go into this, such as cold soup, porridge, cold vegetables or odds and ends of any kind, and tinned or fresh tomatoes make it more savoury. Tomatoes may be cleaned, put in a pie dish, batter poured over and then baked and are very tasty in this way. Butter adds to the flavour of these dishes, but does not make them more wholesome or more nourishing.

'To make a sweet batter, mix wholemeal flour, milk and one or two eggs together, add a little sugar and cinnamon and it is ready for use. Stew ripe cherries, gooseberries, currants, raspberries, plums, damsons or other ripe fruit in a jar, pour into a pie dish; pour over the batter named above, bake, and this is a good substitute to a fruit pie. Prunes can be treated in the same way, or the batter can be cooked in a saucepan, poured into a mould, allowed to go cold and set, then it forms wholemeal mould, and may be eaten with stewed fresh fruit. Rusks, cheesecakes, buns, biscuits and other like articles as Madeira cake, pound cake &c can all be made of wholemeal flour. In making the wedding cake used at my marriage "breakfast", wholemeal flour was added to the other ingredients. Wholemeal flour thickens soup, or you can make wholemeal soup thus: chop fine any kinds of greens or vegetables, stew in a little water until thoroughly done, then add plenty of hot water, with pepper and salt to taste and, a quarter of an hour before serving, pour in a cupful of the batter named before and you get a thick, nourishing soup. To make it more savoury, fry your vegetables before making into soup.

'Substantial bread puddings are thus made: soak crusts or slices of brown bread in hot milk or hot water, crumble fine in a pie dish, add to this soaked currants, raisins, chopped nuts or almonds, a beaten up egg and milk, with sugar and spice, and bake in the oven. Or tie the whole up in a pudding cloth and boil. Serve with the white sauce named above, or eat with stewed fresh fruit. These puddings can be eaten hot or cold; labourers can take them to work for dinner, and their children cannot have a better meal to take to school.'

Porridge

Another of Allinson's favourite foods was porridge – one of the reasons, he believed, that the Scots were such a tall and healthy race:

'Porridge is made by mixing the meal of any grain with water and then cooking the mixture. The best known porridge is that made from oatmeal, and is usually boiled. We can make a porridge from the meal of any farinaceous food: from wheatmeal, barley meal, maize meal, hominy, semolina &c and it need not be boiled, but may be cooked in the oven. Gruel is made from finer meal and is not so thick as porridge.

'The meal from which porridge is made may vary from fine to coarse; when it is desired to make this kind of food quickly a fine meal must be used, as boiling water acts more quickly on the finer particles than the coarse and sooner cooks them. For invalids and children a fine meal is preferable, because porridge made from this kind is more capable of being easily and thoroughly digested than that made from coarser meal. But for healthy adults, and when time is no object, and a finer flavour is desired, a coarse meal should be used. The time that porridge takes to digest depends upon the fineness of the meal and the length of time it is cooked. If made from fine meal and well cooked, it is very quickly and thoroughly digested; but if from coarse meal and not well cooked, then it takes longer to digest and stays a person proportionately. This is why labourers and those who have hard physical work to do find that a coarse and not too-well-cooked meal suits them the best.

'The ways of making porridge are many. The Scotch dribble meal, usually that from oats, into a pan of boiling water, with the left hand, while with a wooden spoon they stir the mass with the other. In this way meal is gradually added until the mass is like thick gruel; then it is boiled and stirred until nearly solid. The additional cooking makes the grains of meal swell and become drier as they increase in bulk. The Scotch use a medium meal and cook the porridge for twenty, thirty or even forty minutes, adding a little salt during the boiling. Unless it is freely stirred in the cooking process, that part at the bottom of the pan gets burnt, and the reason for dribbling the meal in is to prevent particles from caking and forming uncooked lumps of dry oatmeal. Some mix the meal with water at night and let it soak twelve hours, and then cook it about a quarter of an hour in the morning. And some put the coarse meal into a jar in the oven, add plenty of water, and let it cook for two or three hours. All these plans are good. When there is very little time for cooking in the morning, the latter is the best, for, being prepared the day before, it only requires heating to be made ready for a meal.

'Crushed wheat, barley, maizemeal, hominy and semolina, or mixtures of any or all of these can be made into porridge in any of the ways described. The coarser the meal, the more cooking is required. Porridge may be taken at any meal, or a good meal may be made from it alone. The Scotch formerly had porridge at every meal, and did not tire of it. If we weigh out a portion of meal and make that into porridge, we find that the meal has absorbed about four times its weight of water. If milk is taken with this, a very sloppy mess is formed in the stomach, digestion goes on slowly and waterbrash, or the rising of water into the mouth, results. For the same reason, tea, coffee, cocoa or other fluids should never be taken with a meal at which porridge is eaten.

'I find the following way of making porridge very good for those with weak digestions: mix milk and water in equal parts in the porridge pan, add the meal, but no salt, and cook until stiff. This should be eaten cool without milk or salt, but with a little wholemeal bread to make sure of it being well mixed with saliva. Those who are costive may eat a little stewed fruit with the porridge or fresh fruit afterwards. The practice of taking sugar, jam, honey, preserves or treacle with porridge is bad, as these cause acidity, heartburn, and other troubles. Porridge may be taken cold as well as hot, and in summer cold porridge makes a very pleasant meal. Oatmeal or maizemeal may be used in the cold months, and wheatmeal or barley meal in the hotter ones. From a dietetic standpoint porridge is good, as it is made from good material and simply cooked; and, not being mixed with spices, condiments or sauces, is easy of digestion. All classes may eat porridge with benefit, and if the precautions and rules I give are attended to, good results must follow its use. Children thrive on it and grown-up persons keep well on it at very little cost.'

Celeriac

One of Allinson's favourite vegetables was celeriac. In his essay *Celeriac or Celery Root*, he decried the fact that it was hardly ever eaten and most people didn't even know what it was. Sadly, it is still the case today that celeriac is a rarity, even when in season and often only found via specialist organic suppliers. When it is found, though, Allinson was right – it is quite delicious:

'He who makes two blades of grass grow where only one grew before is a benefactor to mankind; and he who invents a new dish is worthy of a place among the gods. So said the ancient Romans. To introduce a food new to this country or to most of my readers is the object of this article. Celery root, or celeriac as it is called by gardeners, is a root not unlike a swede turnip in appearance and it has the flavour of celery. It is well known in Germany and largely used by the Germans as a vegetable for the table and in salads. In both cases it is boiled before being eaten; when put in salads it is sliced like beetroot. This root is good in cases of rheumatism, gout, stone, and diseases of a like nature and is very useful as a food in cases of eczema and other skin diseases; it is also a good anti-scorbutic. It can be used in many cases where beetroot, on account of the sugar it contains, is inadmissible and it can be eaten freely by all as a pleasant addition to our few winter vegetable foods. It will be much better for us physically if this root is on our tea tables rather than winkles, shrimps or tinned fish. As a nation we eat too gross animal foods and too few vegetable products. The use of this root as a regular food will improve our health, temper and condition. One great advantage about it is that it will keep good until April or May is far advanced, and so supply us with a vegetable at a time when the ordinary ones are out of season.

'**Cultivation**: The seeds of celeriac can be got from any large seedsman or florist. These should be sown early in April in a slight heat under glass or under a hand glass on a warm border and afterwards pricked out or transplanted like ordinary celery. About the middle of June the plants should be planted out on the level ground, in moderately rich and rather sandy soil, in rows about eighteen inches apart, and each plant should be a foot away from the one next to it. Before planting out, most side shoots and side roots should be removed. The plants should be put shallowly in the ground and plenty of water given. Occasionally a little of the soil must be taken from round the root and side shoots removed. When nearly full grown a little earth should be drawn round the root to completely cover it, and make it whiter for the table. The roots will be ready for use in September and October.'

Milk (good) and Butter (bad)

'Cow's milk is the secretion found in the udder of the cow and is meant for the sustenance of the calf until it can eat and digest grass. It begins to be secreted before the calf's birth and its production goes on until the calf can live on grass only. In a state of wildness, the calf may suck for about nine months, but in civilised places the duration of the milk secretion may be prolonged to eighteen months or even two years. When milk is drawn from the udder of the cow into some receptacle, it is found to be of a whitish colour, rarely with a tinge of yellow, has an odour peculiar to itself, a slight fatty and sweetish taste… . Out of ten parts of milk we find that eight and a half are water, even if none has been added by the milkman. When milk is examined under the microscope, it is found to consist of a whitish fluid in which small particles of fat are found floating. When milk is allowed to remain undisturbed in a vessel, a yellowish scum rises to the top; this is cream. From it butter is made by churning. When milk is kept in any receptacle and exposed to the air, it soon goes sour, as germs fall into it from the air, cause fermentation and then the curd separates from the whey. This is known as the lactic acid fermentation.

'How long it is since man learnt how to milk cows and use the milk as a food is unknown, but the time must have been very remote. When used with certain precautions, milk is an invaluable article of diet for persons of all ages. It must never be forgotten that milk is a food and must therefore be taken as a food rather than as a drink. For this reason, it must never be taken between meals, if only thirsty, or for supper instead of cocoa. If this rule be disobeyed, then stomach troubles may arise, just as much as if extra meals were eaten. If the animal from whose udder the milk is drawn be diseased, then the milk will be inferior or contain some of the disease germs from which the animal is suffering. Or if the milk has been mixed with impure water, or put into cans which have been mixed with impure water, it may contain the eggs of worms or the germs of disease. Or if there is any kind of fever among the inmates of the farm from which the milk came, some of these may fall into the milk, multiply, and cause a like fever in those that drink it. Outbreaks of scarlet fever have been thus traced to the supply of infected milk from a farmhouse where scarlet fever was raging among the children. To prevent milk being injurious from any of the causes given, it must always be boiled and then the disease germs in it are killed and the milk may be taken with safety.

'When using milk as food, we must take it properly. We may learn this from nature and observation. If we watch the calf, we will find that it has to suck the milk slowly, and in sucking a certain amount of saliva gets mixed with it. If we want the milk to lie light upon our stomachs and to be easily digested, we must sip it slowly and mix it with saliva. I always recommend milk drinkers to sip the milk very slowly, or even to take it from a teaspoon; then it does not curdle in the stomach in heavy masses... .

'The value of milk as food is that it contains nourishment in an easily digestible form, and those who are used to meat and wish to adopt a non-flesh diet will find the free use of milk very helpful whilst making the change. Sickly, weak and delicate persons will find milk a valuable food if they will use it as I advise and growing children may take it very freely, but only at meal times. When babies cannot get breast milk, then that of the cow mixed with barley water must be given. Breast-fed children, when weaned from the bosom, must be allowed milk and bread, or milk and some farinaceous food if old enough. As children grow older, they may still use milk freely; at meals they should drink it mixed with water instead of tea or coffee. They may also have porridge and milk, or brown bread and milk sop at least once a day. Grown-up persons will also find milk puddings advantageous.

'During illness or recovery from disease I find milk an invaluable food. In disease of the stomach and bowels I rely almost entirely upon milk and barley water to keep my patients alive, whilst the necessary curative changes are proceeding. In ulceration of the stomach, a diet of milk and barley water only is the best cure. Equal proportions are mixed of each; a tumblerful is allowed every four hours; the mixture is slowly sipped when cool... . In all fevers and inflammations, or acute illnesses of any kind, I nearly always keep my patients on milk and barley water until the worst symptoms have passed. By means of it, I can keep down inflammation and prevent complications better than drug doctors can with their poisons, and my patients are not injured by the milk as they are by the medicines. In acute disease, put the patient at once on a cup of milk and barley water every four hours until the doctor comes. This mixture is far superior in value to all the beef teas, beef extracts or animal soups ever invented. It alone will sustain patients for weeks during sickness, for a patient will get well quicker on cold water than he will on beef tea and such inferior and injurious extracts. For the future, I ask my readers to use milk and barley water as their sheet anchor in disease and they will never repent of it.

'It is best to use milk in its entirety. Cream, butter and cheese, being products of milk are not so good as the entire article. Butter and cream I condemn, because they are they are only the fatty parts of milk. Cheese is a fairly good food; it consists of the fatty and nitrogenous parts of the milk solidified and preserved with salt. It should be used sparingly and thoroughly well mixed with other foods, else it is apt to be indigestible and cause trouble... .

'Another good way of using milk is to cook it with farinaceous foods and make puddings with it. Rice, sago, tapioca, hominy, macaroni or some such farinaceous food should be steeped or soaked in water until soft, then milk poured over and the whole baked in the oven. When milk and egg are beaten up together and baked in the oven, we have what is known as a custard; this must be used sparingly as it is a concentrated food, liable to cause biliousness, congestion of the liver and an upset of the stomach... .

'Skim milk is a good food, and those who are inclined to stoutness or skin eruptions may use it, as the cream has been taken from it. Buttermilk is also good, and may be used under like conditions but it is more fattening. Those who are inclined to put on flesh must use milk in all forms sparingly. Curds and whey are good food. Milk is curdled by means of rennet or even of a bruised nettle put into it. The whey may be drunk as a cooling drink, with or without a little lemon juice. The curd may be eaten with bread or stewed fruit. In Germany sour and curdled milk is very popular. It is thus made: milk is put in tumblers or shallow dishes, and allowed to stand in a warm place for twenty-four or thirty-six hours. At the end of that time the milk will be quite sour and almost solid and the cream is on the top. This may be eaten with dry bread at breakfast, lunch or tea time. Sour milk need never be wasted, but allowed to set, and then eaten as I advise. Every consumer of milk should test their milk by letting a little go sour in a tall glass. If the milk will not curdle, it shows that soda, borax or other chemical has been added; these make the milk unfit for use. If water has been added to the milk, it will separate on souring and show at a glance that we have been buying watered milk. Another test for milk is by means of a clean polished knitting needle. It must be dipped in the milk and immediately withdrawn; if the milk clings to the needle it is pure, but if it runs off and leaves the needle nearly dry, suspect that water has been added. Then try the souring test, and if both show added water, change your milkman, or report him to the Medical Health Officer for your district. For the future I hope readers will use milk wisely; it is more nutritious than beef tea or any alcoholic drink, and is an excellent food.

　　'NB: If too much milk is taken or if the person who uses much of it is inclined to rheumatism, he may suffer rheumatic pains from its use.'

Chapter 4

WHAT NOT TO EAT
– OR DRINK

HAVING EXAMINED the list of Allinson's perfect foods, it is clear that many of the ingredients of most popular present-day diets are entirely missing. And Allinson did, in fact, have a very long list of foods that he would happily ban. Some of them have been found today, more than a century after his recommendations were regarded as ludicrous, to be the cause of many health problems. Take salt, for instance – or rather, don't:

'During the Nineteenth Century before refrigeration, salt was widely used as a preservative and, as a consequence, many people consumed a great deal of it. This was not thought to be a cause for concern amongst the medical profession. Allinson thought otherwise:

'The practice of salt-eating is almost worldwide. No doubt, first started as an accident or peculiar taste, it spread, and is now kept up like many other evil things, because it has the sanction of usage and antiquity. The habit of eating salt is an acquired one, as any one may judge for himself if he will only give it up for a time and then try to take it up again. Animals in a natural condition will not usually eat salt, nor will the untutored savage. Civilised man has accustomed himself to eating salt, but he is no better for so doing but, on the contrary, is injured by it. It is related of Peter the Great that he tried to accustom his sailors to drinking salt water instead of ordinary water, so that they might not die of thirst when at sea, but his experiment failed and many died during the trial as a consequence.

'Common salt, called by the chemist chloride of sodium, is a mineral widely distributed all over the earth and is found more or less in all water, but more especially in sea water. It is part of the mineral matter of most plants and of the fluids of most animals. Being thus found in the mineral, vegetable and animal kingdom, I may be asked my objection to its use, seeing also that it is usually a constituent of the tears and the urine. My objection to salt is that it is a mineral and therefore should never be used. Man is not fitted for directly absorbing mineral matter and if he takes such material either as salt or in the form of medicine, he must do himself harm. The only way that man may take common salt or mineral matter is when it forms an actual and organic part of the food that he eats. In other words, the fruits, grains and vegetables contain all the salt necessary for our systems, and if we add more, we err and do to ourselves an injury. The fact that salt is found in all our tissues and fluids is no argument, for the greater part of it got there after being added to the food. Again, if no salt be eaten and yet it is found in our systems, we must know it comes through our food and is kept in the system for the body's use. One might as well argue that because ashes are found in the fireplace, the fire must therefore be fed with ashes, as that because salt is found in the tissues, you must therefore eat salt. Persons who eat brown bread, green vegetables, salads and fruits obtain from these foods all the salt required by the system. A human being has no more cause to eat common salt than he has to eat phosphates of lime, iron, manganese or any other mineral. The blood and tissues contain all these salts in solution, but that fact does not make it a necessity for us to eat them in their mineral form. Our system will abstract all it requires if we will only give it some of the proper foods before named.

'What results follow if we do eat salt? They are many and varied, but I will only mention a few of the more evident. Salt stimulates the appetite, causing us to overeat and from over-feeding come seven-tenths of our ailments. In the stomach salt causes acidity and heartburn. That it irritates the stomach we all know, for salt and water is a common remedy used to make a person vomit. Salt being very soluble in all fluids is quickly absorbed by the vessels of the stomach and taken into the blood. As a consequence it thickens the blood, makes it denser than it should be and causes the sensation called thirst. To quench this, fluids must be taken. If only water is consumed, then digestion is delayed for half an hour and the kidneys have to do more work. If tea, coffee, beer, or other injurious liquids are drunk to quench this thirst, then we must suffer from diseases produced by these fluids, besides overtaxing the said organs... .

'Some one may ask, are there no diseases which will arise if we do not take salt in our food? To this I answer none; no disease can arise as a consequence of abstaining from salt. I may be reminded that prisoners were said to be devoured alive by worms in the prisons of Holland, because the persons in authority stopped their salt. This I at once brand as an historical lie. I can never find any authentic authority for it; it is an antique lie, but none the less a lie. Against this statement I can bring forward fact such as this, that I know living persons who for years have carefully abstained from salt in everything. Then salt does not prevent worms, neither tape worms, long worms, nor thread-worms, nor do standard books of medicine advise salt eating as a preventive against them.'

While salt was on his list of banned substances, other minerals were not. In the essay that follows, *Saline Starvation*, Allinson explains the importance of mineral salts and where they are found naturally occurring in foods:

'I now propose to tell my readers how they waste much valuable mineral matter which their systems require and how they may remedy this. We find that the usages of society prescribe that foods shall appear in certain forms or of certain colour; to attain these conditions foods are broken up in various ways and only parts of them put on the table to eat. Very few foods reach the table as prepared by nature, but are disguised in various ways, altered, but never improved.

'Mineral matter is required by our systems to build up the bones and the teeth, and also to keep the blood of proper consistency so that it may obey well known mechanical laws. The want of mineral matter from the blood is very injurious and many diseased conditions of the body thus arise. In childhood, absence of mineral salts in the food leads to rickets or softening of the bones. This rickety condition is the cause of bowed legs or pigeon chests and of water on the brain. If a child does not get food containing a fair amount of mineral matter it is backward in cutting its teeth and in walking; and if this condition of things continue, then the body remains short and stunted instead of remaining a proper height. The decay of women's teeth during pregnancy and suckling is explained thus: her offspring requires bone-forming material for its bones, and as the mother does not eat enough mineral matter in her food, the system takes it, what it can from her bones and teeth to nourish the child and the consequence is that the mother suffers and the child more or less as well.

'Other results of deficient mineral matter in the blood are various skin diseases. The scurvy, at one time a very common complaint, and now not uncommon, was brought about entirely by the absence of mineral matter in the blood. Fruit and vegetables soon cure it. Any sailor can testify to this. Eczema and other skin eruption often arise from the same cause and are cured by fruits, vegetables and green stuff. Gout, rheumatism and hardening of the cartilages round the joints and other places are due to excess of lime salts. These diseases arise because the foods men eat are tampered with, certain salts are left in them that the system cannot well use and so remain in their bodies and cause trouble by being deposited round the joint, as sand or stones are about projecting rocks or windings in the rivers.

'How does this saline starvation arise? I answer, chiefly by the mutilation of foods and secondly by cookery. The mutilation of foods is seen when we grind wheat and throw away the bran, which contains nearly all the mineral matter of the grain. Also when we eat fruits without their skins. Cookery has much to answer for; when vegetables are boiled, the water dissolves out the soluble mineral matter, which is lost when the water they are boiled in is thrown away. This is the evil, what is the cure?

'**Cure**: This is simple. First, do not throw away the bran, nor separate it from the flour, but grind the entire grain as fine as you can, and use that as food…. When eating fruits do not throw away the rind…. The skins of cucumbers, tomatoes and vegetable marrows may be eaten, also the skins of roasted potatoes. When vegetables are cooked they should be steamed rather than boiled, as steaming does not dissolve out the mineral matter as boiling does. A very little trouble is needed to make our present saucepans into steamers. Rivet two hooks into the pan near the top, opposite each other, swing a wire basket from these; and cook your vegetables in this. A small quantity of water at the bottom of the pan will generate enough steam to cook with. If these directions and rules are adhered to, my readers will not suffer from saline starvation, nor will they need to add much salt to their food to give it a flavour, in place of that which has been lost in the cooking.'

The Demon Drink

Of course, it was not only salt that was used to make meals more palatable. Wine, beer and spirits were drunk in quantity – and even believed to have beneficial effects on the health. In Victorian times, in fact, wine in particular was regarded as having medicinal properties. Dr W Lauzan-Brown, a former sub-editor of the Lancet, in his *Useful Information for the Home* recommended burgundy for convalescence, anaemia, debility and loss of appetite; claret for its 'powerful action for good' on the digestion and nervous system; port for preventing colds and chills; sherry for exhaustion of the brain or heart; and champagne for ladies, convalescents and invalids.

Allinson, of course, took a diametrically opposite view – that they were in fact poisons. 'To have the best health,' he thundered, 'alcoholic liquors must not be taken,' explaining he wrote from an entirely medical and scientific – not moralistic – point of view (and it was, of course, the time when the temperance movement was a major force). In *Why People Drink*, an essay in his first collection, he examined the underlying causes of the demon drink:

'In most parts of the so-called civilised world the use of certain stimulating liquors is common. Most people use them (some more than others) and it is my wish to examine the why and wherefore of this and note the results. In the first place we must presume that people drink because they know that fermented drinks produce well-known effects on the system. If we analyse these liquors we find that they all contain a chemical compound known as alcohol. It is the action of this compound that we must study. We must study its action on the body just as we would any other drug like opium, mercury or prussic acid. It is a poison and as such should be kept only in chemists' and doctors' shops and should not be sold as freely as it now is, for anyone to buy who has the necessary money. Its common and almost unprohibited sale accounts for its frequent use, for we find that the more places there are for its sale the more is used of it.

'Food satisfies the craving called hunger, alcohol does not satisfy the craving called thirst, but tends even to make the thirst greater. One reason why some people drink is because they have a craving for it, which craving was born with them. Their parents were drunken and they have given this craving of drink to their offspring. Their drunken parents may have three or four children. One likes drink, another is an idiot, another has fits and so on. Other people drink to satisfy an inward craving or emptiness they feel. This emptiness is brought about by wrong kinds of food, which fill the stomach, but do not satisfy the wants of the system... . Overfeeding in the same way produces a desire for alcoholic drinks; these drinks act by paralysing the stomach nerves for a time and so pain is not felt. Breathing bad and vitiated air sometimes produces a low feeling, to cure which stimulants are taken. Many drink to drown care, trouble or sorrow or even to lessen joy. They do not like to face worry of any kind, so they stupefy themselves with drink and put off the evil until a later day. Many drink from want of occupation. Thus, people with means which place them above the necessity of working, drink to fill up the spare time. Many drink because their occupation takes them amongst drink; such as barmen, potmen, waiters, brewers' men, travellers for wine merchants and nearly all men connected with the drink trade... .

'Many drink from want of a comfortable home. Thus, a hard-working man comes home from work and finds it in an untidy state, perhaps with no food for him, no fire &c. He naturally goes to the public house, where he finds congenial companions and an obliging landlord as long as he has any money. In this class we must place the young men with fairly good educations, who go into large towns to earn a living. Office hours are over say, at 6pm, and having nothing much to do, they drop into hotels for a drink and a chat, or play billiards and drink until the habit grows on them. They little know the chains they are fastening on themselves or the physical evils, the seeds of which they are sowing.

'Some drink to try to keep warm, like cabmen, sailors &c. Drink certainly gives a feeling of warmth, though it does not produce warmth, in reality it cases a lowering of the heat of the body. Some few drink to cure pain, to relieve indigestion, sickness, wind or diarrhoea. Simpler remedies than intoxicants can be used without producing ill after effects... .'

Having laid out the underlying causes, Allinson goes on in the next essay, *The Results of Drinking*, to discuss the repercussions:

'The effects that are seen after alcohol is taken are due to the system trying to get rid of it. One of the first results is an increase in the number of the beats of the heart. The heart usually beats about 72 times a minute, but a moderate dose of alcohol will increase this up to 100 or 120... . Dr B W Richardson has shown that one ounce of alcohol will make the heart beat 3000 times more than it would have done if no alcohol had been taken. This represents, in figures, a weight of three tons being lifted a foot high by the heart.

'An ounce of alcohol is contained in two glasses of beer, two glasses of wine or a glass of spirits. Taking this as our basis of calculation, we can readily see how a single glass of beer taken daily for ten, twenty or thirty years must exert an injurious influence over the system. What must be said of those who drink many beers, wines and spirits every day? My readers can now understand why I am continually advising persons to abstain from all intoxicants, for they waste life and lay the foundation of disease. I am also against their use in illness, because they lower vital activity and instead of doing good, they do mischief and make the chance of recovery smaller.

'Another result is the dilatation of the small blood vessels or capillaries of the skin. This causes a feeling of warmth, which is unreal, as the heat of the body is actually lessened. This dilatation explains the flushing of the face that some experience after a single glass of wine and accounts for the red faces of those who are habitual tipplers. On the brain alcohol exerts an influence like chloroform and ether. That is, it is an anaesthetic. It paralyses the brain centres which control the action of the muscles, as we may judge by the unsteady walk, trembling hand, difficulty of speech and double vision which are experienced by persons under the influence. The reasoning faculties are also disordered. From this arises the proverb, "When wine is in, wit is out" for a man then reveals secrets he would otherwise keep to himself and commits indiscretions which he would not do in his sober moments.

'The blood is also acted on injuriously by this agent. Alcohol prevents the red corpuscles from carrying a proper supply of oxygen to the tissues. The blood does not get thoroughly aerated and so waste is retained in the system, which waste is the cause of many disorders from simple pimples on the face and body to gall stones &c... . The organs which get rid of alcohol from the system are the skin, lungs, liver and kidneys… . But every organ it comes in contact with is injured and if this goes on, last disease is produced and death.'

Allinson goes on to describe those diseases in his next essay, The Diseases Produced by Drink. Characteristically, he does not mince his words:

'I must preface this article by again saying that alcohol is a poison like prussic acid, strychnia, arsenic or phosphorus and if taken daily for a long period of time produces grave diseases… . Among the mildest complaints produced by alcoholic drinks we may mention vomiting and sickness if more than a certain quantity is taken. Stomach complaints are very common amongst drinkers, such as flatulence and distension from decomposition of food in the stomach; whilst dyspepsia and indigestion are nearly always found to follow the use of alcohol, on account of the hardening and thickening influence on the stomach… . The more grave diseases of the stomach produced by alcohol are gastric ulcer, cirrhosis or thickening of the stomach and lastly cancer… .

'After the stomach, the next organ to be affected is the liver. Here, congestion and hardening are produced. There is a hardened condition of the liver known as hob-nailed or gin-drinker's liver. Congestion of the liver gives rise to piles. The countenance becomes sallow in persons with obstructed and congested livers. The whites of the eyes become yellow and jaundice may result. Gall stones are also produced as a secondary result. The kidneys are affected by this poison and a very serious complaint brought on – that is chronic inflammation or Bright's disease… . The heart is weakened, the blood vessels become hardened and a fatal disease known as aneurism produced. This hardening of the arteries of blood vessels is known as atheroma and this state is usually found in persons who have a fit of apoplexy or a stroke as it is commonly called… . We find in connection with alcohol drinking many skin diseases… . Those on the nose are very properly called 'grog blossoms'… . In consequence of waste being retained in the system, gout and rheumatism are very prevalent among drinkers. One of our great London physicians – Sir Andrew Clark, I think – said that from 75 to 80 per cent of the persons seen in hospital owed their presence their to drink.'

In the final essay in the series, Cure for the Drink Crave, Allinson recommends an improved diet, tepid bathing, fresh air and giving up all other stimulants such as tobacco, tea and coffee. And as replacements for the demon drink? 'At dinner, lime or lemon juice and water is good or fruit juices mixed with water. A drink that nursing mothers can take is thin gruel, cocoa or milk. Herb drinks are not to be despised; such drinks are nettle, dandelion and herb drinks, ginger beer and some few others.'

The sweet – and blackened – tooth

It was not until the Nineteenth Century that sugar became cheap enough for most people to afford it. From Tudor times onwards, sugar had become very popular at court – Queen Elizabeth's teeth were black by the end of her reign – but by Victoria's reign, it was used by every level of society. Allinson wrote: 'Sugar is an article of diet so widely used that to write against its free use will be looked upon as foolish, yet this is what I propose to do… . Fifty years ago its price was too high for it to be commonly used and it was only brought out on state occasions. Even now in Belgium it is too dear for free use by the labouring classes. In Germany instead of making fruit into preserves with sugar, they boil the fruit down into a thick, porridgy mass and use this in place of jam… . Millions of people in this and other countries have lived, loved, married and died without ever having tasted manufactured sugar… . Only we who live in the age of manufactures and so-called advanced civilisation know what it is to eat artificially prepared sugar and to suffer from its too frequent use… .

'When sugar is consumed in its natural form in ripe, raw and fresh fruits it is a good food; it is also natural when it is formed from the starchy foods we eat. It is not so good when eaten in dried fruits as in dates, raisins, figs or currants, as it is out of proportion to the other constituents; and when taken from the cane or beetroot and purified it will be found more or less injurious to everyone.

'Babies who are fed with milk sweetened with sugar suffer from wind, griping and purging… . Babies are also made cross, irritable and fretful from the presence of sugar in their blood… . Children who eat much sugar are apt to suffer from all kinds of skin eruptions as eczema, pimples, boils &c or may be fretful, irritable, restless and nervous… . In adults it is the cause of many complaints; it causes us to overeat; and goodness knows we have too many temptations of that kind. It sets up thirst, which is often quenched with all kinds of injurious liquids; in the stomach it is a common cause of wind and acidity, while bowel flatulence of a distressing kind is often brought on by it… . Stout persons are warned against it as it increases their condition.'

Clearing the lungs

In the Nineteenth Century, it was common medical advice to suggest that smoking a cigar or a pipe, even a cigarette, was beneficial, a way of 'clearing the lungs. This may seem farcical to us now, but at the time there was no link between smoking and cancer. In fact, Allinson was one of the first to suggest that there was one – though not cancer of the lungs. He was violently opposed to smoking on many fronts, as the essay simply entitled *Tobacco* in his first collection explains:

'Tobacco is the dried leaves and stalks of an American plant, the manufactured article having first been introduced into this country by Sir John Hawkins in 1565 and into France by Jean Nicot in 1559. Nicotine, the poisonous principle of the plant, derives its name from its French introducer. Tobacco rapidly exhausts the soil of mineral matter, as the tobacco plant requires much of this for its growth. Good tobacco contains at least two per cent of nicotine. Tobacco is now used by nearly all the peoples of the earth, and to give the results of a study of its action on mankind is the object of these articles. It must never be forgotten that none of nations of antiquity ever used it, and that all the science, philosophy and teaching of the ancient sages, heathen and Christian, were taught to disciples who neither used nor even knew of the existence of this foul poison. Nicotine – the poisonous principle – is, next to prussic acid, the quickest poison we have. One drop of it kills a rabbit in three and a half minutes, and a man has been killed by this poison in four or five minutes. A thirty-second part of a grain given to a man causes alarming symptoms, while a sixteenth of a grain produces bad effects for three days. A single cigar contains enough poison to kill two men. Children have been killed from using a well saturated tobacco pipe which they used to blow bubbles; they absorbed enough of the poison from the pipe to cause death.

'Cigarettes are the most injurious form of using tobacco, as so many are smoked in succession and the smoker also often draws the smoke into the lungs and so more of the poison is absorbed. Boys are also sufferers from cigarette smoking. Pipes are bad, especially when they become saturated with tobacco juice. Cigars are bad and the last inch of them is the most injurious. To chew tobacco is bad, but one of the least harmful ways of using it, as in smoking the burning of tobacco introduces into the mouth ammonia and other injurious products of combustion. This latter fact shows that to smoke herbal tobacco is not good. Snuff is the least harmful of all the ways of using tobacco, but it is the dirtiest; snuff injures the membrane of the nose and causes constitutional symptoms of tobacco poisoning. Tobacco was at one time used as a medicine, but it killed so many and so quickly that its use has been stopped. In asthma its action is unreliable; as a poultice it has caused death. Even habitual users of tobacco have killed themselves by using it immoderately; men have smoked for wagers and have killed themselves by smoking twenty pipes or cigars one after the other.

'We will now study its effects on the various organs. The first indulgence in tobacco usually causes vomiting, weakness, cold shivers and a great feeling of prostration. If its use is continued then it produces other well marked symptoms. The heart is an organ that suffers much; tobacco causes it to enlarge, dilate and the valves are so affected that they do not properly close. It so excites the heart that it greatly increases the number of pulsations to nearly double what they ought to be, that is on first smoking and in seasoned smokers it always increases its action. In time, in consequence of this, it causes an irregular action of the heart; one beat out of five or six being missed – if five or six beats were missed all at once we might die. It also causes dull pains in the heart region and also palpitation. Users of tobacco suffer from rapid beating of the heart and palpitation or excitement more than those who do not use it.

'Users of tobacco are very liable to suffer from anaemia or bloodlessness, as tobacco causes dyspepsia and then bloodlessness results.

'The action of tobacco on the digestive tract is bad; it dries the tongue, mouth and throat, causes congestion of these parts and also ulceration of them. Ulcers of the tongue, throat and even of the stomach are often seen in tobacco slaves and caused by it. Smokers' sore throat is a well-known disease. Speaking, singing, and swallowing are interfered with by the use of tobacco; the tonsils enlarge, catarrh of the throat is set up, and smokers do not get rid of a cold so quickly as those who do not use tobacco. Tobacco causes more saliva to be poured into the mouth; when this is spat out thirst is caused and drink of some sort taken. Temperance reformers state that smokers break their pledge in greater numbers than do non-smokers. The saliva of smokers is not so strong as it should be. Dyspepsia, catarrh of the stomach, and many other digestive disorders are caused by tobacco. The more expensive the tobacco, the more dyspepsia is set up. Smoking blackens the teeth, and causes tartar to be readily deposited on them. At first tobacco causes purging, but after a time it helps to set up constipation.

'Cancer is often due to the use of a pipe; it frequently arises when the pipe rubs and if a person is liable to cancer then the irritation of the pipe may start it off. When this fell disease once comes it is difficult to cure. Most of the cases of cancer of the lower lip are found in smokers. Women rarely smoke and rarely suffer from cancer of the lip. Tobacco does not cause lung troubles, but when a cold is caught the smoker does not recover very quickly as a rule, whilst a cough is always made worse by it. When a person suffers from chronic disease of the lungs we find that tobacco increases the quantity of phlegm.

'On the muscles its action is bad; it causes weakness, tremblings, want of proper control over the muscle and helps on or causes paralysis of the legs. Athletes should never use it, nor should engravers, lithographers or those who do fine work of any kind.

'On the nervous system its action is well marked. It causes timidity, loss of energy, indecision and want of will power. It causes nervousness, tremblings, blushing, bashfulness, flushing, vague foreboding, sleeplessness, lowness of spirits, irritability, twitchings of the muscles during sleep, cramp in various parts and paralysis. In France it has been noted that the increased use of tobacco is followed by an increase in the number of insane persons. It causes or helps on blindness, loss of hearing and of taste and smell. Specks before the eyes, ringing noises in the ears, and sudden attacks of giddiness are caused by it in some. It increases the perspiration. In the young it upsets digestion and nutrition and stunts growth; also causes heart disease and impairs the memory and helps on many nervous disorders.

'Smokers will suffer from some of the following symptoms: loss of appetite, coated tongue, constipation, foul breath, restlessness, sleeplessness, nightmare, irritability, morbid fancies or ideas, paleness, sallowness, thinness, colic or cramp, weakness, tremblings, stomach troubles, disorders of sight etc. Wounds in smokers do not heal so readily as in those who abstain from it.

'The best way to stop this injurious habit is to give it up suddenly; there will be great craving and a feeling as if something were lost for four or five days, then the natural man will predominate and health and comfort be gradually restored.'

Corruption of the flesh

Allinson was a vegetarian for almost of all his adult life and he proselytised enthusiastically about it. He believed that little nourishment came from eating meat or fish and that they brought with them unwanted side effects, as he suggested in his essay *Popular Fallacies about Flesh*:

'There are a number of fallacies floating about the country concerning flesh food, and as many of the delusions are popular and widespread, people on that account often believe in them. My purpose in writing this article is to destroy some of these delusions, by relating the full facts of the case. The first and greatest fallacy encountered is that meat, or the flesh of animals, is a necessity for man. Three-quarters of the world's inhabitants rarely touch fish, flesh or fowl, but draw most of their nourishment directly from the vegetable kingdom. The flesh of animals contains nothing that cannot be got better and cheaper from fruits, grains and vegetables. Flesh is only grass, or other vegetable matter, second hand, and as for being the essence of vegetable substance or concentrated vegetables, it is not. On the contrary, flesh is poor in sustaining qualities and contains little nourishment. Meat consists of nearly 12 oz of water in the pound. A pound of peas, beans, lentils or macaroni, is equal in food value to four pounds of flesh meat and one pound of these foods will give more force to the body for hard work than four pounds of flesh will. Let my readers try the experiment and flesh will lose its hold on their minds as being a food of much value.

'After solid flesh we will consider meat soups and essences. These are regarded as being very nourishing, in fact they are looked upon as if they contained all the nutriment of meat in a small space. This is another delusion. Beef tea, mutton broth, chicken broth, rabbit broth, veal broth, shin of beef soup and all the rest of the animal soups and broths contain very little nutriment. They contain less nutritious matter than an equal quantity of milk and a good deal less nutriment than an equal quantity of well made wheat meal porridge. For soups to be at all nourishing, they must be thickened with barley or other grains or vegetables. As for meat essences, they are more than useless, as they contain waste matter of all sorts, which floods the system with stuff it cannot use. The use of animal broths and meat essences in sickness will tend to keep the person ill longer than if he never took them at all. As for oxtail, turtle and other like soups, they must all be put down as very poor and very high priced articles of diet.

'Oysters are reckoned very nourishing and light of digestion. This is not so, they only contain about a fifth of their weight of food, or even less than that. Therefore, to get nourishment from oysters you have to pay more than from 5s to 15s a pound for it and then it is inferior to that got from good wheaten bread. As for being easy of digestion they take as long to digest as any other raw flesh food; that is, about three hours. They are swallowed whole, and therefore by not being properly chewed, they take longer to digest than well-masticated food. That they do not lie heavy or cause inconvenience, is because they are taken raw, in small quantities, and usually without other things to upset the stomach. Let other foods be taken in the same way and more good will be got. As for stout and oysters combined being nourishing and restoring, the reverse is the case. The simplicity of the oyster meal is upset by the stout, which more or less coagulates the albumen of the oyster, and makes it harder to digest; the stout also delays digestion by precipitating the pepsin or active principle of the gastric juice, besides inflaming and weakening the stomach.

'As for chicken, lamb and poultry being light foods, they take, on the contrary, even more time to digest than plain beef or mutton and are not one bit more nourishing. Lastly, we have fish fallacies, that fish is good brain food, or that it is a lighter food than meat. It is not a better brain food than meat, does not contain more phosphorus, but it is a little easier of digestion as it contains more water, and is, therefore, more easily broken up by the gastric and other juices. For brainwork it is inferior to wheatmeal bread, which really contains phosphates in abundance. If such fish as salmon, eels and mackerel are eaten, then the effect is like eating fat meat, as their flesh contains so much oil. Weight for weight, fish, flesh or fowl, contain less nutriment than good wheaten bread.'

The beastliest beast

Of all the flesh foods, though, Allinson reserves his greatest disgust for pork, which he regards as unfit for human consumption in an essay entitled *The Pig as Human Food*:

'The Germans have a proverb to the effect that "A man is what he eats" and if we apply this to the subject of our article we may say that a pig is what he lives on. We know from practical experience that the pig eats dirtier food than any animal; no filth is too foul for him. Abroad where he can roam about in the forests, he eats wild nuts, acorns, and a variety of ground nuts; but as a whole, the pig is a dirty feeder. In the country pigs are fed on swill, which is composed of dish water, scrapings from plates, potato peelings, apple peelings and refuse of all sorts. Rotten potatoes, rotten apples, waste of any kind is given to the pig. When he is being fattened he is fed on fat-forming food, as peas meal, barley meal, Indian corn meal and buttermilk; but before fattening on refuse of any kind. In towns they are not fed so well as in the country. I have seen them in a knacker's yard eating the entrails and refuse of dead horses: and there is a story on record of one pig-keeper contracting for all the old poultices from a hospital – this I have on good authority. I have seen pigs root up the buried entrails of a fowl and eat them greedily. In America I have been told they will follow cattle which have been fed on corn, and eat their excreta for the undigested corn in it.

'The pig cannot be called the scavenger of the world, as man eats him, and so becomes the scavenger himself. This animal is not clean at home, his sty is very often ankle deep in decaying straw, mixed with his own droppings and urine. His exercise is limited to a few feet or yards each day. His life may be said to consist of eating refuse, sleeping and making fat out of the stuff given. His skin is dirty and scurfy, rarely getting a wash, and altogether he leads a most unnatural and unhygienic life. The consequence of this improper living is a diseased body; the pig of civilisation may be said to be in a state of chronic disease. To try and clear the system from impurities nature establishes six or seven small running sores in the fore feet on their inner surface. It is very unusual to find a pig without them and it is not an appetising thing to remember than when we eat bacon or ham we are eating part of a case whose feet were ulcerated.

'In consequence of the dirty feeding habits of pigs they are often infested with parasites. That most to be dreaded disease, trichinosis, is derived from the pig. This animal eats refuse in which the eggs of the parasitic lurk; the trichinae are set free in his stomach, migrate into the muscles by the thousand and produce what is known as measley pork. If man eats of this, and if every part is not thoroughly cooked, he brings on himself this most terrible disease and one for which we doctors can do nothing. It is common in Germany and we have had some outbreaks in this country. The tapeworm of the pig, or that got from eating its underdone flesh, is more difficult to get rid of than the beef or mutton tapeworm, as it has a circle of small hooklets on its head by which it attaches itself to the intestines, and so hard to dislodge. In consequence of plenty of food and little exercise the pig soon becomes fat and were he not killed when he is, he would die from apoplexy or from fatty degeneration of the heart. Fat animals are diseased animals, be they cows or pigs and he who eats their flesh is eating waste or disease that their systems could not get rid of.

'Now what is the result when man eats of the flesh of this dirty animal. In the first place the flesh of the pig, called pork, is very hard of digestion. It takes from five to six hours to digest, and thus uses up a great deal of vital energy which could be used for other work; ordinary lean beef or mutton only takes three hours to digest. For his reason only very strong persons can eat pork without being upset. Pork being rich in fat, causes acidity of the stomach, heartburn, indigestion and bilious attacks. In some cases it gives rise to acute dyspepsia and vomiting. If eaten for supper it causes nightmare, horrible dreams and sometimes even death.

'The Shakers, as a community, found after they left off eating the flesh of pig, that cancers and tumours were less common among them. The morning rasher that people eat is taken chiefly for the salty flavouring and is a most unhygienic food. The insipid white bread that many people eat wants something to help it down, and so salt bacon is called in. Would people eat brown bread they would need no relish with it. Tobacco, alcoholic liquors, spices, condiments, sauces, mustard, &c, destroy the taste, so that ordinary foods are said to be flavourless or tasteless without them. Consequently strong tasting foods, such as pig's flesh must be eaten or else they have no enjoyment from their meals. For myself I live so simply that lard in pie crust almost makes me sick, and pig in any form or shape I have not tasted for many years. Looked at from a scientific and practical point of view, no person who values his health and his life can afford to eat pig in any form, be it bacon, ham, pork or sausage.'

The cup that cheers?

While Allinson's convictions as a vegetarian and general healthy liver make his distaste for meat and tobacco understandable, one might expect him to take a kindlier view of drinking tea. In fact, it too gets short shrift and, as a committed cocoa man, Allinson lays bare its faults:

'Tea is a beverage that is used greatly in the United Kingdom, in our Colonies, in America, in Russia and in China. The question arises in many minds, has it any injurious properties? Some would laugh at the idea of tea doing anyone harm, which nevertheless is the case. To properly study the question we must look at it from many sides. We must ask ourselves – 1st, is the tea pure; 2nd, if not, what are its adulterations; 3rd, its temperature when drunk; 4th, the constitution of the person who drinks it; 5th, is the stomach empty or full at the time it is drunk; 6th, the time when the tea is drunk.

'Before looking into the question in detail, I must make this positive statement, that tea of itself has no nourishing properties; in other words is no use or value as food. Physiologists tell us that it prevents tissue waste: they mean that it prevents the waste material in our systems being thrown out; if it does so, it must do harm. As a beverage the only nutriment a cup of tea contains is the sugar and milk that are added; and it is far inferior to cocoa, or to milk which are foods. The injurious effects of tea-drinking are due to the alkaloid of tea theine, to the adulterations, and to the temperature of the water drunk. The theine, which is the active principle of tea, and a nerve poison, causes more or less paralysis of the heart and unduly excites the whole nervous system. Tea is thus shown to be a nerve irritant, causing first a feeling of stimulation and vigour, but leaving dullness behind. It fills the mind full of ideas; but they are visionary ones and not practical.

'Persons who drink very largely of it are often brown, thin and shrivelled up. To many it is an actual poison and they do not know it. Let any person give it up for a time and then take a cup of fairly strong tea and note the results. He will find first pleasurable excitement and rapid ideas, which are followed by trembling of the whole body, wavering over work, indecision, a want of confidence generally; and a frontal headache is the final result.

'Tea is the great cause of indigestion, especially if strong, as the theine of the tea throws down the pepsin from the gastric juice and so prevents its action. If a meat tea is taken, the tannin or bitter part of tea hardens the fibres of the meat and prevents it being dissolved. When the tea is absorbed by the system it causes more or less wakefulness, as it is well known, for persons wanting to keep awake drink strong tea. Those who are restless at night may take a hint and never drink tea in the evening. It affects the heart's action, causing unnecessary excitement of that organ. Its action on the nervous system is bad, as it tends to cause palsy or loss of power over the muscles. Men have been tea-drunk and staggered about as if drunk from spirits. These are the chief effects. All persons who are nervous, timid, shy, or who suffer from loss of energy, want of memory, will power, or of firmness of character, should avoid it. Its action on the reproductive system, especially of men, is bad; and it causes loss of manly vigour more than many drugs.

'The adulterants used in making tea look good are injurious; they are chiefly salts of iron; sometimes Prussian blue, black lead &c. When much adulterated the tea-drinker has to suffer two evils instead of one.

'The last part of our subject is the temperature of the water with which it is made. If the tea is taken scalding hot, it causes loss of taste, cracks the enamel of the teeth and relaxes the throat. In the stomach it causes congestion, and if disease is present, sets up violent pain at once. If a healthy person habitually drinks hot tea, coffee, cocoa, or even hot water, he weakens his stomach and makes it irritable, besides which the bowels become of an inflamed tendency and diarrhoea and colic are set up.

'Much tea is one cause of a red nose or red eruption on the face. If the stomach is full when the fluid is take, it delays digestion for some time. In summer, hot tea relaxes the pores of the skin and makes a person perspire very much. Those who drink tea must not take it hot, but should wait until the heat has nearly left it, and drink it only lukewarm. The habit country people have of pouring the tea into their saucers is good; it is not fashionable, but it is more healthy than drinking it scalding hot… .

'To sum up, tea drinking is injurious and should never be indulged in; all are best without it. Never have it strong nor hot; never drink it near bedtime; never take it if going to do fine bodily or mental work of any kind and do not give it to children at all.'

This lukewarm – in every sense – approval of tea is not extended to beef tea, a favourite Victorian drink for the weak or recuperation after illness:

'One of the most popular fallacies in this country is about the goodness and sustaining properties of beef tea. It is supposed to be the sheet anchor in disease, and as long as people get it they imagine they are taking one of the most nourishing and satisfying foods possible. Never was there such a mistake; beef tea is one of the poorest, least nourishing and least sustaining of foods and far inferior to gruel or to milk. To show the truth of what I assert, plain facts shall be given. Before doing so I may state that our medical papers have shown up the fallacy again and again, yet doctors still order it, and sick persons still look to it as a good food.

'There are two kinds of beef tea – first, that made from the extract which is usually sold in pots at a fabulous price; second, that made from fresh meat. In making the extract seen in pots, they say it takes forty pounds of meat to make one of extract, and many imagine that it contains the goodness and strength of these forty pounds. Instead of containing any goodness it contains all the refuse or excrementitious matters which would have been thrown out by the kidneys in a few hours if the cow had lived. As the British Medical Journal puts it, beef tea thus made has much the same composition as urine – a pleasing idea this. In making this extract all the fat is skimmed off and away goes the heat and force-forming matter. The flesh is then boiled and the juice strained off, the flesh being afterwards used as manure and thus the muscle-forming part of the flesh is thrown away… .

'The next kind of beef tea is that made at home from fresh lean beef. This is cut fine, put in a jar; this is placed in the oven, and in an hour or two a tablespoonful or so of thick fluid is poured off, which forms a jelly when cold, and this is supposed to contain the nutriment of the pound of flesh. It is very little better in nourishing power than extract, as this jelly has been found by experiment to be capable of giving very little force or heat to the system… .

'Doctors often order beef tea because they think it nourishing, or else because they would lose their patient if they did not. When I wish to lower a patient I order him beef tea; but if I want to nourish him, I order it to be made with barley, rice carrot, turnip, onion &c. These are they that supply the necessary nutriment and not the beef… . In sickness I always order a gruel made from wheatmeal, oatmeal or rice, sago or tapioca, with milk. When soup is desired, beef or bones may be used as a flavouring, but I always tell my patients to add lentils or peas, pearl barley or rice and some celery, onion, carrot, turnip or other vegetables.'

Allinson had, as ever, strong views on all forms of drinks. In his essay *Thirst* he explains that, ultimately, the only proper drink is water, though he does have a few others that he doesn't completely condemn:

'As hunger is caused through the system wanting nourishment, so thirst is caused through the tissues requiring fluid. The body is composed of solids and fluids in the proportion of three parts liquid to one solid. In other words, if we take a body weighing a hundred pounds and dry it thoroughly, we shall find that it weighs only twenty-five pounds, the rest having been water. We are continually losing fluid in many ways. However dry the food we eat, the undigested part of it always passes out of the body, saturated with moisture. However dry the air we breathe, it returns from the lungs quite moist. This we can see for ourselves very readily; breathe on a glass or on a cold polished surface and a deposit of moisture occurs. The skin is daily losing a large quantity of fluid as insensible perspiration, and the kidneys usually get rid of two or three pints of water in the twenty- four hours. Altogether we lose five or six pints of water in the twenty-four hours in the natural condition. During violent exertion we lose more fluid by perspiration and by the breath, and less by the kidneys.

'Thirst is a demand of the blood and tissues for fluid, so that they can carry on their work. Water is the only thirst quencher, and the purer it is the quicker will it fulfil its purpose. It only is what the tissues demand. After water, thin cocoa, lemon, bran or barley water and herb drinks are the best thirst quenchers. Milk, thick cocoa and all stimulating fluids are not good for this purpose. Alcoholic drinks allow one to have the satisfaction of drinking without materially quenching the thirst.

'The back of the throat is the part to which we refer our sensations when we are thirsty. This is due to the fact that the back of the mouth has a surface very well supplied with blood vessels, from which moisture is always exuding or being secreted to keep these parts moist. When the blood is thick and does not contain its usual quantity of free fluid or if it be laden with much salt or sugary matters, then it does not allow much of its liquid to escape and the throat becomes dry and we feel thirsty. Thirst is thus seen to arise from an absence of free fluid in the blood, or to that state in which the free fluid holds in solutions sugar, salt or other saline matter. That thirst is due to the blood and tissues craving for water, we can prove in two ways. If we drink water we can quench our thirst, or if water be injected into the veins or tissues it is relieved. On the contrary, if a tube be fastened into the gullet of a dog so that the fluid drunk passes over the throat, but is not taken to the stomach, but allowed to pass into another vessel, the thirsty dog will drink for a long time without abating its thirst. Thirst is a symptom of disease in diabetes. It is then due to the blood containing an undue quantity of sugar.

'**Moral**: Those who do not want to suffer much from thirst will use salt and sugar in great moderation. They will also avoid salted, peppery and seasoned dishes. Fruit and salads, grains and vegetable foods do not cause so much thirst as do animal foods or products. The vegetarian suffers much less from thirst than does the mixed feeder. When thirsty, water is the fluid to drink; the purer, it is, the sooner will the thirst be allayed.'

And when not to eat ...

Allinson not only had strong views on what to eat and drink but when to eat and drink them. In particular, he believed eating late at night would do no good at all:

'A supper may be defined as a meal taken a little time before going to bed. Three meals a day are enough for anyone and he who takes more does himself harm. These meals should be so arranged that the last one is at least three hours before bedtime. Those who do night work must not take a meal immediately before going to bed in the morning. Some are so circumstanced that they find it almost impossible to get an evening meal, except just before retiring. In cases like this, supper must be both light in quality and small in quantity. Those who work hard after their tea meal must not make this an excuse for eating when that work is done. Actors, speakers, lecturers and those who keep their business places open until late should never take suppers; the hard work they have done is no excuse. Some say they cannot sleep unless they have a meal just before gong to bed. On inquiry you will find that the slumber or unconsciousness that they do get as a result is not that sounds refreshing sleep that a healthy person enjoys.

'You may ask, why do I object to suppers? I answer: for two reasons – first, because of the physiological results; and secondly, because of the ill effects that experience shows are a consequence of these late meals. During sleep, waste of the body is actively got rid of, and repair of the various tissues takes place. From five to seven hours is the natural length of time required for the healthy person to sleep. In this space the necessary tissue changes occur, the muscles rest, and are then fit for another day's work. If food is in the stomach when we retire to bed, that food must be digested before proper sleep can come. Digestion takes from three to five hours, according to the food eaten. Milk puddings take two to three hours; beef, mutton fish and other plain meats take three or four hours; while cheese, pork, ducks, veal, ham &c, may take from five to six hours to digest. Let us take three people and give them a supper at 9pm, say they go to bed at 10.30pm, and have to get up at 6.30am. The first one has a milk pudding; this takes two and a half hours to digest. Number one gets no refreshing sleep until about midnight, will not feel fresh in the morning, but gets up feeling more or less heavy. The second has some meat; his real sleep will not come on till one, he only arises with great effort, and feels anything but bright. The third one has some pork or cheese and pickles for his supper. He does not fall into refreshing sleep until about 2am. When 6.30am comes he is sleeping heavily, is aroused with difficulty, scarcely knows where he is, dresses mechanically, and is half asleep for an hour or two.

'What does experience show is the result of suppers? It proves that supper eaters either fall into a heavy sleep which is accompanied by nightmare or troubled sleep, or the person dreams that he is occupying himself all night by doing over again the work of the day. Or he tosses and turns in bed, dozes off, but wakes with sudden twitchings of his limbs and does not sleep properly until the food has passed from his stomach. Supper eaters are bad risers in the morning. When they do get up they have very little energy or inclination for work. They feel tired, their mouths taste nasty; they have no desire for food, and they are often disagreeable and disgusted with themselves and everything else. It is only after being up two or three hours that they recover their self-composure. Troubles peculiar to young men are made worse by suppers.

'**Summary**: Avoid food for at least three hours before going to bed; better still, four or even five hours. A cup of cocoa is the best refresher to take after a heavy night's work, not milk nor solid food. Those who wish to rise early, be risk and lively and get refreshing sleep, will avoid the late meal. A walk of half-an-hour just before going to bed helps on good sleep.'

PART TWO: HEALTH AND SICKNESS

Chapter 1

SURVIVING THE VICTORIAN DOCTOR

THE LONG-RUNNING wrangle that was Allinson's relationship with the General Medical Council was deep rooted. There are, though, some question marks over exactly what those roots were. One of the causes cited by the medical authority was that he was endorsing and selling products (his flour and other wholemeal items) and that this was improper for a doctor who had to be seen to be above commercial interests. However, Allinson believed his 'infamous professional conduct' was perhaps more to do with his views and advice that were put forward in no uncertain terms in his widely read column in The Weekly Times and Echo.

Victorian England was not a healthy place. Almost half of all children failed to live to the age of five and life expectancy was a mere 43 years. Allinson's 'hygienic medicine' proffered a new way of looking at the nature of health and disease, one that rested mostly on self-help. By means of diet, exercise, fresh air and other ideas that are now so widespread as to seem simplistic, he believed the nation's condition could be improved beyond recognition. This in itself was regarded by the rest of the medical profession as pretty cranky but his advice that smoking was harmful was outrageous at a time when most doctors recommended a cigar or a cigarette as an excellent way of clearing the lungs. However, he went further still and condemned his colleagues as doing more harm than good, using drugs that were useless at best but more likely harmful to the patient.

With hindsight – and knowing the content of most of these 'medicines' – it is clear he was almost entirely in the right. However, as he realised, his views were not shared by the vast majority of doctors and they were quite prepared to close ranks against his unorthodox ideas. In one lecture he summed up his colleagues thus:

'There are 25,000 of us in the United Kingdom, and we stick together more closely than any other profession. You may take the Law or the Church, and you will find in neither the same intense devotion to corporate interests. If one makes a mistake, the others are ready to hide it. Many coroners are medical men, and when a case occurs that is not favourable to the profession, it is more or less dexterously slurred over. By means of this trade unionism we have acquired immense power, which is yearly increasing. Law and Church will soon be accounted second and third. People cannot be born without us; they cannot die without us; and it will come to pass that they cannot be married or take a situation without us.'

All of this can hardly have endeared him to the medical profession. However, over time it became clear that his views had validity and by the time of the First World War, wholemeal bread was recognised as beneficial and Allinson was offered the chance to register again as a doctor with the General Medical Council, though he refused. He continued to offer 'hygienic medicine' as a way to better health and if many of his opinions today may look like a statement of the obvious, at the time they were regarded as eccentric, outrageous and sufficiently unprofessional to result in his being struck off.

Hygienic medicine

In his second collection of essays, Allinson explained the underlying foundation of his ideas: in a nutshell, that by living in accordance with the laws of Nature, mankind avoided most diseases, whereas by adopting the 'civilized' diet, lifestyle and medical practices, illness, decrepitude and death were sure to follow. In a series of essays, *Natural Conditions, Bodily Changes, The Healing Power of Nature, Unity of Cure* and *Stop Drugs*, he outlines the rules for a healthy life – and upsets his professional colleagues – in one fell swoop. In his preface, he cites particularly *The Healing Power of Nature* as a cause of 'censure of the Edinburgh College of Physicians – to which body I belong' but continues 'the impartial reader will find a plain statement of facts that he can test at any time. If the treatment of disease by drugs is not scientifically correct, then the sooner it is replaced by a safer treatment the better.'

The first essay in the collection, *Bodily Changes*, begins with some basic physiology:

'There is a common saying that the body changes every seven years; the fact is that the body changes every moment of our lives. The system is never two minutes alike, but is continually renewing its structure. I can best show this by giving a few facts about ourselves. Man is composed of millions of very minute particles or cells, whose functions are to keep the body in the form we see it and in the condition of health. Our bodies are composed of nerve cells, muscle cells, fat cells, liver cells, stomach cells, saliva cells, tear cells, kidney cells &c, &c, &c. Each of these varieties has its own work to perform and can do nothing else. Thus the tear cells always secrete tears and the liver cells always secrete bile and so on.

'All these are kept alive and in proper condition by the blood. This fluid contains millions of minute bodies called the blood corpuscles; they are kept alive and replenished by the food we eat and the air we breathe. The blood cells carry oxygen from the lungs to every part of the body, so that the tissues may use it to allow force to be generated and for change and repair to go on… When every cell has taken up its oxygen and nourishment from the blood it throws into it all its waste. This impure blood is conveyed to the lungs and purified by them, as well as by the liver and kidneys. After this cleansing it is fit again to start its round. Certain cells are thus seen to be scavengers, as those of the liver, kidneys and in part those of the lungs… .

'Every movement and the performance of every function causes a usage of food. Thus, every thought I think, every breath I take and every action that goes on, uses up food… . The body is continually renewing its structure, cells are always dying, and if were not so replaced by new ones, the body would soon decay... .

'**Moral:** The moral to be drawn from these remarks is that if we wish our bodies to be in good condition, we must supply them with food which will nourish all our tissues in a proper manner and we must not give them material which will famish them and cause them to die slowly of starvation or will kill some cells outright... . I am continually writing 'time and correct living are required for cure'; now my readers can understand why, for time and pure blood are necessary to effect the healthy changes we desire.'

In his next essay, *Natural Conditions*, Allinson goes on to explain how, given man's physiology, it should be nourished for optimum health – however demanding this may be:

'Many persons look on me with disfavour because I tell them to conform to certain rules to obey which is sometimes a little troublesome. These laws are as immutable as those which govern the sun, moon, stars and the rest of Nature. I am only an interpreter who tells his audience what is his reading of these laws.

'My readers should always remember that man is physically an animal only and nothing more; I want everyone to recollect this and not to imagine that he is something special. He is only an animal like a horse, elephant or monkey, but with a higher intelligence; and is subject to exactly the same natural conditions as they are, for if these animals live under wrong conditions, like man, they suffer in exactly the same way... .

'I classify [man] as a fruit and grain eater, therefore my advice is always tending to vegetarianism; for I find the best health can only be obtained under this system of diet. I ask people to avoid rich, greasy, fatty and sugary foods because experience has shown how very injurious they are. I ask them to avoid suppers, because we find those persons who take food in the evening, within three hours of retiring, are never so well as those who avoid a late meal. Three meals a day only are found best to agree with our present conditions. Eating slowly and chewing well are demanded by our teeth and stomachs, so that digestion and absorption may be properly performed. To stop as soon as satisfied is demanded by the system, for if we eat after this warning the surplus food takes away energy and by flooding the system with excess is the starting point of disease. It is also a fact that man does not always want the same amount of food; our system knows when to demand more and when it can do with less and makes us to know this by the feeling of satisfaction that is set up.

'Man being an animal requires pure air; this is why I so persistently ask my readers to have pure air everywhere; to keep their sitting-room, work-room and bedroom windows always open, even in very severe frosty and foggy weather, as such cold or muggy air is more beneficial than hot bad air... . Exercise is another necessity of our existence, especially if we want to enjoy life to the fullest extent. Our various muscles were intended for obtaining our food and if we do not exercise these we come to grief; two hours a day will keep us off the sick list, more will give us robust health. Bathing is demanded because we wear clothes which retain the perspiration and because in bathing we expose our skins to the open air to which in nature they would always be exposed.

'Secondly, I object to stimulants and narcotics. In a state of nature, alcohol is always a product of rotting fruit and is never found in the concentrated form of rum, gin or whisky. Thus, if a person tried to get drunk on rotten apples or pears he would be deterred by the acrid flavour of the decayed fruit from so doing. Experience has also shown that alcoholic drinks are great disease producers. Tobacco also, on the same principle, is a poison that only repeated use makes us tolerate and, like alcohol, is a poison that gives rise to much ill health. Tea and coffee are nervine irritants, as anyone can prove for himself if he will only give them up for a time and then note the ill results on again taking them. These are my reasons for always advising the same rules and why I object to alcohol, tobacco, tea, coffee and other poisons. I try and interpret Nature's laws to my readers; again I say, I am not the author of these laws, which all must obey if they wish to live well.'

It is no doubt the views that Allinson expressed so forcefully on drugs and the other medical practices of the day gave most offence to his colleagues. In *The Healing Power of Nature*, he explained why he opposed them so strenuously:

'I am constantly asking my readers and patients to stop drugs; some few then want to know how they will get well if they take no medicine. So far I have simply required them to follow my advice; now

I give them reasons why they should take no physic. First, I must tell them that all curative and healing power is inherent or natural to the system; secondly, that disease is generally a curative process and when an upset occurs, the body is curing itself and setting all to rights. To those who are living wrongly disease is thus a most salutary process; it clears their systems for the time being of all waste material, for they tell you, 'I was better after that illness and in better spirits than I have been for years'; and if they have sense enough, it warns them that they have been living wrongly… .

'The healing power of nature is a stored-up vitality, by means of which we recover from illness and accidents. Let us suppose a man cuts his finger and if he does nothing to it – not even wrap it in a piece of rag – will that finger get better of itself? Certainly, and quicker if left alone than if meddled with. This healing power first stops the bleeding by shutting or blocking up the mouths of the divided vessels… . Next, from the cut parts, serum, or the colourless fluid of the blood, is poured out; this forms a seal over the injured part, fresh cells form, new blood vessels and nerves shoot into the part and in a time varying from one to two weeks, the part is whole and entire, with only a little scar to show where the cut was… . From this example we see how Nature heals and it leads me to ask, What is the result if we treat wounds with various ointments &c? In many cases the results are bad. If we use carbolic acid lotion, we may destroy some of the growing cells and retard healing besides; the carbolic acid may also be absorbed by the system and give rise to symptoms of poisoning. Such cases have occurred again and again… .

'Are we in good condition, then our wounds heal quickly; are we in a bad state of health, they heal slowly. Too much meat, too little exercise, bad air, dirty skins, the use of tobacco and the drinking of beer, wines and spirits, produce a low form of vitality and the results are lingering illnesses and slow recovery from wounds and accidents.

'Let us study a case of simple fever: the pulse is 120, the tongue furred, the bowels costive or relaxed, the urine scanty, high coloured and throwing down a thick sediment; there is severe headache, feverishness, thirst, loss of appetite, distaste for food, sleeplessness &c. If we leave such a case alone, will Nature cure, and if so, how? She will readily do so, more especially if right conditions are observed. In the first place, the weakness and pains would keep the patient quiet, so that the system could use all the strength for curative purposes; next, the distaste for food, and even the occurrence of vomiting or diarrhoea would prevent for the time such being taken into the system; lastly, free perspiration would throw out of the body impure material and then recovery would take place. The symptoms we see are the result of the fever and of burning up the waste matter in the system, which waste must be got rid of before health can return.

'Man being an animal would, if he were under proper conditions, be out in the open air whilst this was occurring. This is Natural cure. Now how is this process interfered with by ordinary doctors? Very often, instead of giving the stomach rest, they order vile concoctions of grease and waste from some animal, which they call broth and which almost would make a healthy person heave. They then wrap the burning hot patient in heavy bedclothes, order the window to be kept shut, allow no water, but send some poisonous medicine instead. The result is that your patient throws up the greasy broth when given. He tosses and turns in bed, first on one side then on the other, he jumps and starts, and wakes up from horrible dreams with an anxious look on his face, his body burns, his tongue is parched, he feels on fire and the drugs given may increase these symptoms. This may go on for a week or two until Nature cures the patient in spite of doctor and drugs, or else he dies, not so much from the disease as from drugs and neglect of natural conditions.

'On the other hand, the hygienist would act thus: he would order the windows to be kept open a little and a fire kept burning so that thorough ventilation and fresh air would be secured to burn up waste; next he would order two tepid baths a day, to cool and cleanse the surface of the body and assist skin excretion. Cold water would be allowed in plenty and acid drinks if the patient craved for them. The food would be of the lightest, as gruels, simple non-greasy soups, fruit drinks and fruit itself. As for drugs, the hygienist never uses any except as poisons for parasites. The result of this mode of treatment is a comparatively mild attack, quick recovery and few or no complications afterwards. I treat all my cases of fever thus, and get most quick and remarkable cures, be they cases of small-pox, scarlet fever, measles or typhoid fever.

'Inflammation of the lungs, acute pleurisy and bronchitis are to be treated much on the same lines. Nature cures all these complaints if you will only give her proper conditions. Chest complaints always require plenty of as pure air as possible. Stomach complaints, in addition to these conditions, must be treated very carefully with regard to diet.

'Chronic diseases require time; in these, proper hygienic rules and the avoidance of tobacco and stimulants are necessary. Some patients are so worn out that a non-flesh diet is the only one from which they can get any relief. Gout, rheumatism, liver and kidney disease require careful living, with plenty of fruit and green stuff. Syphilis, which is really a low fever spread over six months, must also be treated on the same lines. Mercury, in this disease, is the most disastrous remedy that man ever devised and is the cause of most of the bad results.'

Dangerous drugs

In the two articles, *Unity of Cure* and *Stop Drugs*, Allinson launches his fiercest attacks on the medical profession, advocating 'hygienic living' as the logical alternative to drugs:

'Many persons cannot understand that all diseases require only one mode of treatment. Being brought up to the old idea of things, they imagine every disease requires a different remedy. Thus, when they hear of liver disease, they think of podophyllin, blue pill, &c. If they hear of consumption, it suggests to them cod liver oil, stout and beef tea; for coughs and colds they recommend you ipecacuanha, squills, paregotic &c. For every real or imaginary disease they have a fixed remedy; if the person gets better whilst taking the drug, it was the drug that cured him; if he does not recover, then they try something else. They do not believe that a person can get well without drugs and if you tell them that you successfully treat all diseases without drugs, they then ask you what drugs were sent for... .

'All cure must be based on one foundation, namely strict obedience to the laws which govern health. Many may be astonished when I tell them that the same mode of treatment will cure diseases of apparently different kinds. Thus, whether I am treating gout, consumption, dyspepsia, gall stones, fever, hypochondria, pimples or nervousness, the treatment must be very much the same. One of my readers who did not know me and with whom I was speaking, said I was a fool because 'it did not matter what ailed you, all you had to do was not to smoke, not to drink, to eat brown bread and sleep with your window open.' This man's summing up of my mode of cure was fairly correct. As diseases are caused by bad habits, improper food &c, so cure is brought about by stopping all wrong habits and by adopting correct living, then the system rights itself.

'To get cured of any complaint, except those diseases due to worms or to parasites, certain rules must be obeyed. In the first place all bad practices must be discontinued, such as the use of tobacco, the drinking of beer, wines, spirits and other fermented or alcoholic liquors; drugs, medicines and pills must be stopped; and if any other bad habits are indulged in they must cease before cure can take place. The next thing to do is to put the system under the best condition for the restoration of health... .

'The hygienic rules are also most important aids to cure and as useful as the food eaten. Fresh air is most important in the treatment of diseases, especially those in connection with the breathing organs; thus it is the chief part of the cure and prevention of influenza, cold in the head, sore throat, quinsy, laryngitis, loss of voice, catarrh, cough, bronchitis, pleurisy, consumption and asthma. Exercise must not be neglected, for exercise burns up waste material, improves the circulation of the blood, increases the vitality, strengthens the muscles, enlivens the spirits and gives tone of a lasting kind to mind and body. Bathing cools the blood, cleanses the skin, lessens feverishness, helps to allay congestion or inflammation of internal organs and is in every way beneficial... .

'Very few are aware of the damage done to our bodies by taking drugs which are of no use as foods and which are in plain English nothing but poisons, some deadlier and more fatal than others, but all bad. Many have doubtlessly heard of Mr Gladstone's saying that "drink was more fatal than war, pestilence and famine combined"... . When those words were used, scientific (so-called) medicine was not known. Doctors' medicines were like the old muzzle loading muskets and the new ones like our breech loading guns: the old drugs were bad enough, but nothing to be compared in destructiveness to the simple but more deadly ones now used. The jargon of Medicine (so called

Art) was called by Byron the "Destructive Art of Healing". Doctors killed many, but cured none, those that got well did so in spite of the stuff given.

'Dr Baillie, one of the leading physicians in London many years ago, said on his death bed, "I wish I were sure that I have not killed more than I have cured." … . In fact a druggist, or technically a "pharmacist" gets his name from the Greek *pharmako*, a poison, hence one who sells poisons. If every chemist's shop were decorated with the word 'poison dealer' printed large, what a stir it would cause and yet it would be the truest term to apply to all chemists and druggists; it would be like calling a spade a spade. As it is we call him a poisoner in the Greek language and he takes it as a compliment.

'Every dose of medicine taken is an experiment tried at the expense of a person's constitution. If he survives it is because he has a good constitution which withstands the poison used; if it makes him worse this is often thought to be due to the disease, when it is only a result of drug poisoning. If he recovers in spite of the drugs, then he credits the drugs with the cure and forgets that his system had anything to do with the recovery. Every dose of medicine acts injuriously on the system and instead of aiding cure actually retards it… . Dead men tell no tales; could the dead only reveal what killed them, instead of having on the death certificate "Died from apoplexy", "consumption" or "kidney disease", we should see an immense number of cases thus described 'Poisoned by mercury', 'antimony', 'arsenic', 'morphia', 'digitalis', 'strychnia, 'prussic acid' &c. In other words, it is often the drug which kills and not the disease.

'If there is one subject on which I am bitter it is drugs. If I could dip my pen in a mixture of gall, wormwood, aloes and the strong acids, I could not write in too bitter a manner against them… . Those of my readers who wish to live long must avoid all medicines. If they go to their ordinary doctor, take his advice, but not his physic, and they will recover sooner than if they took both.'

In fact, Allinson went on to devise diets specific to particular diseases and listed them in the Appendix to his second collection of essays as *General Directions in Health and Disease*. The introduction applied to all of the diets:

'**Dietetic** – Have only three meals a day, about five hours apart; eat the food slowly chew it well and stop at the first feeling of satisfaction.

Eat brown bread always and not white. Do not drink more than one cup of fluid at a meal, and that luke-warm and not sweet. Cocoa is much to be preferred to tea or coffee, as it is less injurious to the system. The meals should be eaten deliberately, time allowed for them, and a little rest taken after them, if possible. Avoid fried, greasy foods and such foods as suet, Norfolk and Yorkshire puddings.'

His first diet – 'Ordinary Diet' is mostly to be used as a preventative:

'**Breakfast**: 6 to 8oz brown bread and butter, cup of cocoa; or wheatmeal, oatmeal, hominy or barley porridge eaten with brown bread and stewed fruit.

'**Dinner**: about four ounces lean beef or mutton or of poultry, rabbit or fish; two vegetables always; afterwards a little milk pudding, stewed fruit or fruit pie.

'**Tea**: 6 to 8oz brown bread and butter, boiled Spanish onions, boiled or raw celery or other green stuff, or stewed fruit or milk pudding. Weak tea or cocoa to drink.

'No suppers, nor any food for at least three hours before going to bed, but a cup of cocoa may be taken if thirsty or faint. This diet is for ordinary people, who take the world as they find it, want to keep in fair health and yet not to be deemed peculiar.'

The second diet 'is necessary in cases of heart disease, scrofula and all cases of low vitality, damaged organs or delicate constitutions'

'**Breakfast**: as [Ordinary Diet]

'**Dinner**: thick vegetable soup eaten with brown bread, followed by a milk pudding and stewed fruit. Or a vegetarian pie, or the stew in No 3 Diet. Or simply two vegetables, brown bread and some vegetable sauce. As a second course, milk pudding and stewed fruit. Those who do not eat flesh should sometimes eat peas, beans or lentils.

'**Tea**: same as [Ordinary Diet].

'This diet is for vegetarians, for those who desire to get better health than the ordinary people and for the delicate. It is especially useful in heart, liver, kidney and chronic stomach complaints, in syphilis and in gout and rheumatism. For the hypochondriacal it is the best diet I know.'

The No 3 (or Macaroni) Diet 'is useful in chronic diseases and where the system must be cleared of waste before cure can be expected.'

'For breakfast and tea allow about 4 ounces of brown bread cut into dice, pour boiling milk over this, allow to cool and then eat.

'**Dinner:** 2 to 4 ounces macaroni cooked and made into a pudding; eat with stewed prunes or other fruit. Next day have a stew made of seasonable vegetables, with rice, vermicelli or pearl barley; boil thoroughly, mash them well and flavour with a little salt and pepper; eat with brown bread. Finish up with stewed fruit and bread.

'This diet is useful in all chronic cases, and if kept to for some time clears the body of waste and purifies the image.

'No 4 or (Milk) Diet

'Milk and barley bran or rice water in equal parts; a teacupful may be taken cold every four hours. This diet is a quick cure for violent sickness or diarrhoea.

'No 5 or Fever Diet

'Milk and water, gruel, porridge, vegetable soup, milk puddings, toast water, whey lemonade, bread and milk, fruit fresh and stewed, preserve water &c. These are the foods that should be given in erysipelas, measles, scarlet fever, small-pox, typhoid or other fevers and in acute attacks of sickness of all kinds.

'NB Alcoholic drinks, as beer, wines, spirits and liqueurs are only mentioned to be condemned. Tobacco must never be used by those who wish to be well. All drugs and medicines, patent or otherwise, must be avoided.'

Chapter 2

EVERYDAY VICTORIAN DRUGS

IN HIS fourth collection of essays, Allinson inveighed against some of the most common drugs of the day. His article on quinine, regarded by the medical profession at the time as a tonic, he says, 'In reality, it weakens the heart's action and lessens the power of circulation; it lowers the temperature so that life's changes go on less regularly; diminishes the size of the red corpuscles of the blood and thus less oxygen can enter the system... . Larger doses cause complete deafness, which may be permanent; complete loss of vision and blindness may result, giddiness, headache, staggering gait, great muscular weakness and feeble circulation. Larger doses cause delirium and death in convulsions... . Quinine is mixed with many other drugs as bad or worse than itself, such as arsenic, mercury, iron, valerian, iodide of potassium &c. Quinine wine, iron and quinine tonics and all such preparations are best poured down the sink... . If my readers value their health they will have none of it.'

It seems extraordinary today that arsenic was ever regarded as anything but a poison but in the Nineteenth Century it was ubiquitous. As a pigment it was used in wallpaper, cloth, candles, crayons, toys and sweets. This seems even more incomprehensible when it was used precisely as a poison by suicides and murderers – because it was so very easy to acquire. Allinson gives a graphic description of the symptoms of arsenical poisoning. 'They are burning, in the throat, gullet and stomach, sick feeling and violent and incessant vomiting. The contents of the stomach are expelled first of all and afterwards bile and blood may be ejected with the vomit. Griping pains are felt in the bowels and purging follows. There is intense headache, hot and cold shivers, great depression and loss of muscular power and great prostration. Paralysis, convulsions or unconsciousness may precede death which usually occurs from twelve to twenty-four hours after the poison is swallowed.'

Despite this, Victorian doctors continued to use arsenic as a medicine. Allinson elaborates on its 'medical' uses. 'Fowler's solution is a mixture of arsenic and potash, coloured with tincture of lavender; Donovan's Solution is a terrible mixture of mercury, iodine and arsenic... . Drug doctors prescribe and give it in cases of anaemia or bloodlessness, in skin diseases of a scaly kind as psoriasis and Donovan's solution is given where these are suspected to be of syphilitic origin; it is administered with the hope to improve nutrition, as in consumption; in nervous diseases as St Vitus Dance or chorea; in epilepsy and in neuralgia; also in malarial diseases, as ague.'

It was not just the drugs that Allinson's fellow doctors used that he rejected, he was also against the over-use of surgery. 'It can be stated as a fact,' he declares in *Against The Knife*, 'and proved to demonstration that about three-quarters of the operations which are now performed are unnecessary.' Not only that, says Allinson, they can prove fatal. 'The anaesthetics used to deaden pain while the operation is going on may cause death or the surgeon's instruments or appliances may be unclean in spite of antiseptics, fatal inflammation may follow and death may result through an attempt at remedying some real or supposed trifling deformity.'

In contrast to the conventional medical wisdom of the day, Allinson offers 'hygienic' or 'rational' living and a view that is far more current today than in his own time, in the title of one essay *Prevention is Better than Cure*.

'It is my lot to see a large number of incurable cases of disease. The patients suffering from these incurable complaints must die at no distant date and the only hope I can offer them is that their life may be prolonged and their sufferings lessened. Most of this suffering and premature decay might have been avoided had the persons only known and followed the laws of health. The doctor of the present day is paid for treating persons who are diseased; the doctor of the future will be State kept and his duty will be to keep well, rather than to let them become diseased and then treat them... .

'To avoid incurable disease, we must in the first place avoid intoxicating drinks of all kinds as they are the chief sources of many fatal diseases. Alcoholic drinks inflame the stomach and cause all kinds of stomach troubles from mere dyspepsia to ulceration and cancer; they set up congestion and hardening of the liver, chronic inflammation of the kidneys, fatty or enlarge heart, a peculiar form of consumption and hardening or softening of the brain which may be followed by the epilepsy of drink, madness, imbecility or insanity.'

He further recommends giving up tobacco and doctors' drugs and instead improving the diet, taking exercise and opening the windows. In his following essay, *Health Saving Banks*, Allinson suggests a different way of looking at health:

'Many people in this country are content to live from day to day on what they earn, spend all they make and never put any money for accident or emergency. The result is that when anything unforeseen occurs, they have to starve or go in the union for relief. In the same way many people daily expend all their physical capital; they use up every day the energy and life obtained from their food &c, and if they get a chill or meet with an accident, they are laid upon the bed of sickness and lose both time and money.

'The prudent citizen saves money from his wages and keeps it by him so that if thrown out of work or an accident happens to him, he manages to pay his way by using up his savings. The wise citizen economises his vital force and does not use it all up as it is formed but stores some of it away in his system for emergencies and old age. If he meets with an accident or catches a chill or gets upset, this is only temporary he soon pulls through and is quickly well again; and old age is deferred to a far later period of rest and meditation.

'Unwise men waste their money on things which give little or no return and which they are better without. They create false pleasures for themselves and imagine life is not worth living unless they can drink to their heart's content or smoke as much as they please... .

'Wise men walk when time permits and only ride when urgency demands. The exercise taken and the pure air they have breathed keep them in health.

'**Moral**: Live rationally. Do not waste vitality on things that are injurious to the body, then you will always be ready to meet physical upsets and will escape from many that would carry off less prudent people.'

Chapter 3

VICTORIAN COUGHS AND SNEEZES

ALLINSON WAS, of course, a practising doctor who saw all manner of complaints, including the most everyday ailments that are still without a cure today. He took a characteristically brisk view on how to cope with the common cold that continues to trouble us and even those more serious respiratory diseases that we have finally brought under control.

'Autumn and winter are the seasons for coughs, colds, influenzas and all chest complaints. You can scarcely go into a house without meeting someone who is coughing, sneezing, blowing his nose or speaking hoarsely. In some houses there are graver complaints and persons are ill in bed suffering from pleurisy, bronchitis or inflammation of the lungs. Such diseases are not usually seen among animals in a natural condition. How comes it then that man suffers so much from them? To me the answer is easy. I reply at once that they are produced by impure air.

'Let us compare the habits of the same people in summer and in winter. In summer we find they go out daily, often take walks or sit on the lawn or in the garden, and take their work with them, or they may witness cricket or lawn tennis matches. They also ride, drive and are much outdoors. Their sitting room windows are mostly open all day and their bedroom windows a little at night and they get plenty of fresh air all over the house.

'In winter they do not go out more than is necessary, the daily walk is stopped, there are few rides or drives, or only in closed carriages. The cold air is rigorously excluded, windows are shut, and sand bags are used to keep out the cold air, doors are closed and even mats are put at the door bottom to prevent the air coming in that way. The ventilators, if there are any, are closed; the bedroom window is kept shut, and the room is in some cases warmed by a stove or lamp which vitiates the air. In a moderately sized sitting room you will find five or six persons round the fire, with three gases burning, and as each gaslight consumes as much air as three persons, we can easily understand that the air must soon become foul. Many persons sit in this room from 9am until 11pm rarely going out. They then retire to their bedrooms and sleep shut up in these until morn. This process is gone through from the first approach of winter until spring. Only the young folks rush off to skate or play football. If we feel cold, instead of warming ourselves by exercise we rush off to the nearest fire and warm ourselves by it.

'Now I say positively that our coughs, colds, bronchitis etc are not produced by the cold air, but by the bad air we breathe. For we find rooms heated as warm as they were in summer, and yet the inmates are always suffering from colds. On the other hand, we find persons living almost entirely out doors and never having coughs. Also we notice that those persons who look upon fresh air as a necessity, and have it always in their rooms by night and by day, rarely ever suffer from a cold, and only then from breathing the bad air of close rooms, unventilated churches or places of amusement.

'To know if a room is fit to be in, notice the odour. If one comes out of the open air and finds a room smells close, then the air is bad and unfit to breathe. How many persons can say that their rooms are always fresh? I can, for I know the value of pure air.

'Having got colds, how are we to get rid of them? By at once following the advice given to prevent them. Instead of stopping indoors to try to cure them we must go out in the open air as much as possible, breathe through the nose, have the sitting room and bedroom windows open a little and assist the lungs to throw off the disease by making the skin act with warm baths.

'If a cold is caught, its severity will depend on the state of the system at the time. If the system is in a good condition the cold is soon thrown off; but if not, it may turn to a pleurisy, bronchitis or inflammation of the lung; or if neglected and bad habits continued, it may end in consumption.

'Coughs and colds are best left alone and in future we must avoid the cause which gives rise to them. Most people reading this will think I am giving untrustworthy advice, but experience and better knowledge will teach them that I am advocating the best and quickest mode of cure. A tickling cough may often be relieved by sucking a lemon drop, a jujube or a currant lozenge. Pleurisy, bronchitis, inflammation of the lungs and consumption must all be treated by fresh air if successful cures are desired. Cough mixtures, expectorants, narcotics etc should never be used, as they are poisonous and always make people worse. But warm bathing, exercise, fresh air and plain food are safe and permanent ways of curing. Gruel at bedtime, linseed tea, etc are modes of relieving the system by perspiration but a warm bath is more efficacious.'

In another essay, *Chest Complaints*, Allinson suggests breathing exercises as a way of strengthening the lungs:

'An ounce of prevention is better than a pound of cure, so let me advise all persons who are susceptible to lung troubles, or who are weak in the chest or who have consumption in the family, to breathe as much pure air as ever they can get. Consumption can be prevented if this rule is carried out and instead of being our curse – for it is still called in Italy the "English disease" – it will be banished from our midst. Next as to cure: live as nearly as possible by the rules I have laid down in former articles on correct living and at once start a course of pure air treatment. Learn to breathe properly, ie through the nose, as the air is then warmed, moistened and filtered before it reaches the lungs. To the narrow-chested or weak-chested I cannot suggest a more invigorating practice than that of deep breathing. To do this stand up, lift the head up, throw the chest forward, rest the hands on the hips, close the mouth, slowly fill the lungs with air and slowly let it out again through the nose. This exercise should be practised three or four times a day by weak-lunged persons and about six deep breaths taken one after the other each time. This fully expands the lungs, purifies and oxygenates the blood, and does more good in relieving chest complaints than any known drug or invention. Many quack inventions depend for success on the fact that they make you take deep breaths. To ladies I give one fact, viz: that a woman without corsets can breathe one third more air than one who wears such chest-narrowing appliances.'

Allinson takes a similar view about hay fever – more fresh air and a simple diet, preferably vegetarian – but with additional breathing exercises and, perhaps, a holiday.

'The patient must learn to breathe pure air. This may first be done through a respirator lined with wool, which allows pure air to enter the lungs, but keeps out the dust and pollen. A proper respirator must cover both nose and mouth. Best of all, the practice of always breathing through the nose must be adopted. The nose is a natural filter and those who keep the mouth shut and breathe through it, escape many a chest and throat trouble. A sea voyage, residence in town, or at the seaside where the wind blows chiefly from the sea, will do great good and help to lessen the irritation.'

Chapter 4

ENGLISH LEPROSY AND OTHER SKIN DISEASES

S KIN diseases were very common in Nineteenth Century London and Allinson wrote a series of essays on them. The first was Eczema in his first collection and it is still a problem that is controlled, rather than cured, today:

'Eczema is the commonest of all the skin diseases and in some families there is a constitutional tendency to it. It most frequently attacks the young, but no age is free from it. It is more common in winter than in summer, because in winter people get less fruits, vegetables and green stuff; take less outdoor exercise and do not get as much pure air as in summer. Some few have it worse in summer. These eat the same quality and quantity of food all the year round and take little exercise or pure air at any time. In summer they require less food than they eat and the excess makes their eczema worse. Eczema may attack any part of the body. No spot is free from its invasions, but irritation of any kind will determine its locality.

'**Cause**: The causes of eczema are many and may be briefly said to be all causes which supply the system with more material than it can get rid of, or which causes waste to be retained. The artificial causes are chiefly the use of alcoholic drinks, as beer, wines or spirits; next, but in a smaller degree, the use of tobacco. Among the natural causes we find excess of food or wrong kinds of food play a most important part. Excess of food means more than the body requires. This excess has to be got rid of, and is the cause of much disease. The wrong kinds of food are much flesh foods, sugar, honey or fat. Want of exercise, deficiency of fresh air and not keeping the skin pores open, play an important part. We find that persons who eat well and who exercise freely, bathe often and breathe plenty of fresh air, suffer less than those who eat well, but who are indolent, take little fresh air and rarely bathe. Thus eczema is really a warning that we are not living properly.

'**Symptoms**: Eczema may be roughly described as a cracking of the skin of any part of the body with the exudation of a serous fluid. This may form crusts or scabs. It is attended by more or less inflammation and a thickening of the skin or tissues. This mild inflammation gives rise to itching and there is a constant desire to scratch the part, which then makes matters worse… .

'**Cure**: The cure is simple, easily carried out, and sure. In the first place, tobacco and stimulants must be given up. The dinner or supper beer, or the wine and spirits, must be stopped, and the pipe put out for good. Next, proper food must be taken, wholemeal bread must be eaten instead of white, fruit and vegetables must be taken daily, and fresh fruits must be preferred to dry fruits. Much fish, flesh, cheese, eggs, pastry, sugar, honey or cream must be avoided. Lean meat or fish once a day is all the meat food that must be eaten and in bad cases flesh meat must only be eaten every other day. Bad cases of eczema can often only be cured by a bread and fruit diet… . Exercise must be taken daily. Ladies should learn to walk four or six miles a day, whilst men may walk from eight to twelve. Fresh air should be had whenever possible; and the skin should be kept open by a daily dry rub and a weekly hot bath. These means, if properly carried out, will quickly cure. Beware of drugs, they do not cure, but produce other diseases as well. I have some strong words to say about drugs. One case of eczema I saw had been treated with arsenic until the nails dropped off. Others have injured their stomachs and intestines by the arsenic or mercury taken… . If the irritation is great, a little unsalted lard may be rubbed on the part.'

Some of the skin problems that are still around today were somewhat milder, though Allinson's descriptions in his essay, *Pimples and Blackheads*, are rather alarming:

'Most people are afflicted at one time or another with these unsightly eruptions, but they are seen most commonly soon after puberty. These blackheads, pimples, and some other eruptions are classified by those learned in skin diseases under the head 'acne'.

'**Simple acne**: This first shows itself as little, slightly raised spots, in the middle of which a small point of matter gathers. There is a little irritation whilst it is coming. It soon bursts, a little scab forms, drops off and leaves a small red stain. This is seen on the cheeks, forehead, near the angle of the jaw and on the chest and back. As one crop dies away, another forms and so the disease is kept going for a long time if the causes which allow it to appear are kept up.

'**Indurated acne**: In this variety the spots are larger, the area of redness greater and the duration longer; and when they burst may leave behind them a small scar. This variety is seen most on the back and the face.

'**Rose acne**: This variety is commonly known as 'grog blossoms'. It affects the nose chiefly, then the cheeks and forehead. It is seen more in women than in men, and in drinkers rather than in abstainers. It is always made worse by exposure to a keen wind, to the sun, or a warm fire, and hot fluids and foods increase its violence, as will also mental emotion.

'**Acne punctata**: This variety is known as 'blackheads'. It looks as if small grains of powder had been stuck in the skin. It affects the forehead, sides of the nose and is seen on the chest and back. Its course is usually a chronic one. If one of the blackheads be squeezed out, it looks very like a small maggot; it is in reality nothing more than pent-up skin secretion, moulded into this shape by the little bag it is in. It gets black on the top from the dirt which is always settling on our skins.

'**White acne**: This variety is known by the appearance of little oatmeal-like accumulations seen under the surface of the skin. It affects chiefly the face; and when pressed feels as if something hard were under the skin. The matter they contain is pent-up skin secretion. If they attain any size, pricking with a pin and squeezing out the contents soon cures them. The variety is sometimes a cause of worry to men as it often appears on the scrotum and then they worry over it, but there is no necessity to do so as it is a harmless complaint.

'**Oily acne**: This kind is known by the escape of greasy matter from the skin. It usually affects the sides of the nose at the bottom. The skin is then a little redder than usual.

'**Causes**: All these varieties of acne are produced by wrong dietetic and hygienic conditions. They are seen generally about puberty, because then the mode of life changes. The boy often gives up his simple schoolboy life and diet and takes to a sedentary occupation. He eats richer and grosser foods, keeps later hours and may learn to smoke and take stimulants. The girl takes to some quiet occupation, as dressmaking and also eats richer foods. This I believe to be their origin and not, as some make out, to vicious habits. Rich foods of all kinds are a great source of these complaints, such as fat meats, grease of all kinds, butter, fat, suet, cream &c. Sugar also favours their formation, be it as sugar in jam, preserves or sweet things, or too sweetened fluids and foods. Cheese, eggs and honey must be used in moderation by those who wish to escape these diseases. Alcohol in the various liquors, as beer, wines and spirits, lead to their appearance. These come on also from want of air, exercise and bathing as these burn up waste and so prevent them. Various drugs will cause them, as bromide and iodide of potassium, salts of iron &c.

'**Cure**: To promote cure all bad habits must be stopped. Tobacco in all forms must be given up. All stimulants, as beer, wines and spirits must be avoided. Drugs (especially arsenic) must be shunned, even though they are called 'blood purifiers'. Next, good habits must be learnt. The meals must be limited to three a day; pig in any form must never be eaten; meat must only be taken once a day, or even only every other day, and then not fat. I have noticed that vegetarians are much cleaner skinned and fairer of face than mixed feeders. Much grease must be avoided, be it in the form of butter, pie-crust, or suet dumplings; and take care also of fried things. Preserves, jam, honey and all sweets are not good, as they contain too much sugar. Eat your fruit ripe and raw, because even stewed fruit is cooked with sugar and made too sweet. Avoid sweet puddings and sweet drinks, as tea or cocoa, and use as little sugar as possible with anything. Those who have rose acne must avoid all hot fluids. Exercise must be had regularly, six or eight miles a day must be taken by all engaged in sedentary or quiet occupations. Pure air must be breathed always, in the workroom, bedroom and sitting room. Avoid unventilated places of all kinds. A weekly warm bath and an occasional Turkish one aids cure. Leave the spots themselves alone, but the white acne gatherings may be pricked and squeezed out if they get large and the blackheads may be pressed out with a watch-key.'

These skin problems, though, are small fry when compared to the one he calls 'English Leprosy' – also known as psoriasis:

'Psoriasis is really a variety of eczema and is often called scaly eczema. It is an inflammation of the skin attended with redness, a little itching, and the part affected has a scaly covering. It affects all parts of the body, but is mostly seen on the outer aspects, as on the outsides of the forearm and upper arm, and the outsides of the thighs and legs. It appears also on the skin of the head, on the back, chest, abdomen and sometimes on the face. The eruption assumes different aspects; in some it is seen as small spots varying in size from a split pea to a large bean, and in others we find large masses of it from three to seven or ten inches long and three or four inches wide. In appearance it is as if a thin layer of mortar had been spread over a patch of red skin. The crusts or scales have a mother of pearl look about them, and when pulled off a reddish patch of skin is exposed. When the hands and feet are affected the skin in those parts becomes very thick and horny, cracks form and much pain results. When the nails are affected they become thickened, grooved across, and marked with little pits. As a rule there is not much itching with this complaint. It is commonest in those who are in the prime of life and in the extremes of life is seen amongst the old rather than the young.

'**Causes**: In some it seems to show a hereditary tendency, but in most cases it is acquired from wrong living. Alcoholic drinks help on its production; flesh foods, and all rich foods and sweet foods and drink, and fatty and greasy foods do the same. Impure air, insufficiency of daily outdoor exercise, and a dirty state of the skin are favourable conditions for its appearance.

'**Duration**: It may last only a few weeks if acute, but in the chronic form may stay for years, or even as long as one lives, unless proper precautions are taken to get rid of it and keep clear from it afterwards.

'**Treatment**: May be local or general. As this is a constitutional disease, the general treatment is the only rational one, local treatment being only palliative and not lasting. The diet of the patient is the chief thing to be attended to. A non-flesh diet, proper in kind and amount, with obedience to hygienic rules, will usually cure… . The particular foods to be avoided are fat meats, fat or fried fish, bacon, fat pork, butter, cream, cod-liver oil, fried foods, pastry, cake, sweet biscuits, jam, preserves, marmalade, dried fruits, oily nuts, sweet puddings, fruit stewed with sugar and sweet drinks. Milk and water is to be preferred as a drink to tea, coffee or cocoa, unless these are taken without sugar. Bran water is a good substitute for these drinks, and is made by boiling an ounce of bran for half an hour in a pint of water, and strained before drinking. Beer, wines and spirits must be strictly avoided, and tobacco must not be used. At least two hours outdoor exercise of some sort must be taken daily, more hastens cure. The windows must be kept open at least four inches night and day in all weathers. A daily dry or wet rub of the whole body and a weekly warm bath aid cure… .

'I must warn patients against taking drugs whilst suffering from this complaint. Arsenic is the chief drug remedy used; it is a very poisonous one, an sets up violent inflammation of the stomach and bowels, which is often accompanied by great pain after taking food, violent sickness, diarrhoea and intense prostration. I have seen patients with this complaint laid up for three months in bed after a mild course, as it is called, of arsenic. Phosphorus is sometimes given but it causes pallor, thinness, loss of appetite &c; tincture of cantharides, which is sometimes prescribed, leads to inflammation of the kidneys and bladder. Various external applications are used, such as mercurial ointment, tarry preparations, chrysophanic acid, pyrogallic acid &c. In many cases these irritate the skin too much or affect the system in other ways. They are best left alone. Hygienic cure is safest and surest; drug treatment is always dangerous at best.'

Chapter 5

OVER-INDULGENCE: TOO MUCH OF A GOOD THING?

ALLINSON was, of course, a great opponent of rich food and drink and too much of them. He points to this over-indulgence as the cause for many ills, and especially those that affect the digestive system. He lays outs his case in his essay, *Stomach Troubles*:

'Many writers on disease have said that all our ailments come from our stomachs. This is a broad assertion and not entirely correct. That our feeding habits are the cause of a great many of our troubles no one can deny, and a goodly number of people dig their graves with their teeth; still diseases come from other sources than our stomachs. If everyone ate proper foods, they would still suffer from chest complaints, if they did not breathe pure air. If we overeat and obey not other natural laws, we suffer doubly. Overfeeding makes all complaints worse, as it supplies the system with waste, and waste keeps going all kinds of diseases. The broad assertion can be made, that all our stomach troubles and complaints arise from wrong treatment of this organ. We can easily and pleasantly overload it with food, or we may eat too often or surcharge it with fluid. Hot fluids can be emptied into it, or ices and cold things crammed into it. Foods may be eaten that it cannot digest or that are unfitted for it. Medicines, poisons and irritating fluids are sometimes taken into it, set up irritation, and disorder it. When we know in how many ways we can upset this delicate organ, it is not surprising that we suffer as we do, but that we do not suffer more.

'The stomach is a bag in which food lies until it is wholly or in part digested. It is an expansion of the gullet and guarded by two valves. The gullet end is kept closed by a muscle, otherwise the food would return into the mouth, while the bowel end of it has a projection across it that only allows fluids or semi-solid matter to pass over it whilst digestion is going on. The stomach churns the food the whole time that digestion is going on, so that every particle of food has an opportunity of coming into contact with the gastric juice and being dissolved. Only a certain amount of gastric juice can be secreted daily; if we overload the stomach, some of the food remains undigested and sets up irritation or causes pain or diarrhoea. If we eat too often we keep the gastric cells always at work; they become weak and secrete an inferior juice and then indigestion arises. When we swallow too large a proportion of fluid, digestion is delayed until the extra liquid is absorbed. The time taken to absorb this fluid varies from half-an-hour to an hour. If very hot things are eaten, they destroy the ferment of the gastric juice; ordinary fermentation then sets in and stomach flatulence arises. Very cold drinks stop digestion until they are heated up to the temperature of the body which is about 100 Fahrenheit. Tea, coffee, and alcohol delay digestion, as they precipitate the pepsin from the gastric juice and at the same time harden flesh and vegetable fibres. Pepper, salt, mustard and seasonings irritate the stomach, weaken it and cause a more or less sinking sensation if they are habitually used.

'In this article I can but hint at the harm caused by the wrong foods and fluids I have mentioned…. Many ordinary ailments may be traced to their use and I shall no pains to make my readers aware of the fact that many articles of food are slow poisons.'

He also spares no pains when it comes to describing flatulence, in another essay. 'Flatulence is a collection of wind in the stomach or bowels. That which comes upwards may be flavoured by the food eaten,' he declares. 'Flatulence in the bowels is caused by the decomposition of the food eaten. It may be odourless, but is generally foetid and disagreeable. The foods which cause this unpleasant odour contain a sulphur compound, which is broken up by the action of the bile or other intestinal juices. This results in sulphuretted hydrogen or "rotten egg gas" being formed and expelled…. To prevent stomach flatulence, eat less sweet things and drink less sweet fluids, and do not take your foods too hot, and avoid all fried foods. Alcoholic drinks, as beer, wines and spirits, must be discontinued. Improve the whole general health as much as you can, and then flatulence will trouble you less. If you have it, nothing is so quick a cure as plain cold water; drink a tumblerful and if this fails to relieve you drink another…. Do not add bi-carbonate of soda, sal volatile, brandy, ginger or any other compound, as they are not necessary and they weaken the stomach. To prevent bowel flatulency, avoid peas, beans, lentils, cabbage, onions and radishes, or else put up with the consequences. Thorough cooking of peas, beans and lentils lessens their flatulent properties. When flatulence comes on, exercise is the best dispeller; walk it off if you can or rub the bowels with the hands or even apply hot fomentations. Brandy, ginger &c are useless, as the wind in the bowels may be a yard or two from the stomach.'

Allinson gives a similarly robust account of the problems of constipation and what to do about them. 'Constipation,' he opines in his essay of the same name, 'is that state of the bowels in which we do not have a daily laxation: and when this condition continues it becomes obstruction which is a serious complaint. I may state distinctly that this costive condition of the bowels is a curse due to our present mode of living – our wrong dietetic and hygienic habits. The generality of people have no idea what an important part the bowels play in their existence. Most of the cases of languor, lassitude, inaptitude for work of a mental or bodily kind, headache, lowness of spirits and a want-to-be-left-alone feeling are due to loaded bowels: congestion of the liver, piles, varicose veins and consequent varicose ulcers are also frequently induced. In the young we see prolapse of the bowel from this cause; in the adult any tendency to rupture is made worse by it and in the old, apoplexy or stroke is often brought on by straining at stool. Could we trace many attacks of bad temper, indecision and want of energy to their proper source we should find it to be an undue loading of the bowels.'

He goes on to recommend a variety of cures – mostly in tune with Twenty-First Century thinking – including eating plenty of fruit, vegetables, salads and wholemeal grains and taking sufficient exercise. He is, as always, vehemently against the pills, potions and practices that formed the usual arsenal of the Victorian doctor. 'Drugs irritate the bowels and are then thrown off or got rid of as soon as possible by them, and in doing this the food &c is also carried away. The drugs which healthy bowels will not tolerate and which are got rid of by purgation are many – salts of mercury, antimony and other minerals, also vegetable irritants, such as senna, rhubarb, croton oil, castor oil, gamboge, elaterium, aloes &c. The natural waters which purge contain various salts, such as sulphate of magnesia, sulphate of soda and salts of potassium. With a very little consideration of these facts, no one can help knowing that every dose of purgative medicine they take is injurious, and were it not for the purgation they would be poisoned and die… . I add, in conclusion, that all diseases are made worse by constipation, especially those peculiar to women and to young men. Could I make the sale of white bread criminal, I should do more good for my fellow-men than all the laws that have been passed during the last hundred years, but it would ruin pill and patent medicine makers and work sad havoc among doctors.'

In the following essay, he tackles biliousness, putting it down basically to fatty and fried foods, alcohol and pork. Naturally, he recommends a change of diet but he also supports the idea of 'better out than in'. 'In acute attacks,' he advises, 'the quickest cure is to get the stomach to throw off the offending food. This is safest done by tickling the throat with a feather. The next best thing to do, is to dilute the contents of the stomach with plenty of warm or cold water. Two or three tumblers full of water will usually suffice to stop acidity. In severe cases, the patient must lie in bed or on a couch in a darkened room and be kept as quiet as possible. To rapidly recover I do not know of anything so quick as a starve, take nothing but a tumbler full of warm water every four hours until the worst symptoms are past, then take a small basin of wholemeal brad and milk sop, or a basin of wholemeal gruel, these must only be taken three times a day; if feeling faint, then a drink of water will quickly relieve this feeling. Lastly, adopt a simple diet and try to keep well.'

The final essay in the series is *Plethora*. Not a term, or indeed a concept, much known today, Allinson explains not just the ailment but its wide variety of consequences.

'This is a medical term meaning fullness and is applied to that state of the system produced by over-feeding. Persons who suffer from it are known by their full necks, redness of the face and neck, a certain degree of stoutness ad all the signs of having lived well – as it is called. Persons who carry about with them all these marks are envied by some, and in many cases are considered pictures of health. To the critical eye of a doctor these marks are well-known signs of disease. It is from this class we get most of the cases of plethoric disease (ie disease due to over-feeding and drinking). Such diseases are gout, kidney disease, stone in the bladder, heart disease, cancer and apoplexy. In this class of persons are found the cases of sudden death the public so often read about in the papers. We hear of so-and-so being in the best of health one day, and a few days after he is dead; or we hear of sudden deaths of persons who looked remarkably well quite to the day of their death. These have no reserve vitality. If they should be exposed to the depressing influence of a chill they may get a severe attack of pleurisy, or an attack of inflammation of the lungs or bowels and die. An ordinary person in a fair state of health, if exposed to the same chill, would have had a cold and nothing more. This state is brought about by eating too much food (ie eating more than the system can burn up or use). Alcohol in the form of beer, wines or spirits, helps to induce it, since it causes waste to be retained in the system. Want of exercise, bad air and the daily use of tobacco all tend to aggravate this complaint. The rational cure for this state is to cut down the excessive foods and drinks, and to obey all the rules of health... .

'A commoner kind of this complaint is seen in every day life and is felt more or less by all. I refer to the complaints known as the dumps, blues, being hipped, depressed &c. Some call it the liver, others say they are nervous, some call it indigestion, whilst some put it down to general or nervous disability... . Everything seems to have gone wrong and future prospects look very dismal. They take a morbid view of life, wonder why they were born, and think it would have been better had they never lived. To these mental troubles are added bodily pains. They ache all over, have pains in the back or in the right shoulder, up the neck to the back of the head, the head feels sore and the eyes ache. They have no energy, they feel too tired to walk, and cannot concentrate their brains on any mental work. They want to be alone. If a friend drops in and engages their minds on some lively topic it banishes this feeling for the time. It is whilst in this state that many persons commit suicide. I have known a lady start off to drown herself whilst in this condition, but the exercise necessary to get to the water, which was a couple of miles away, took away the low feeling and she returned home cured for the time.... When an attack comes on, the quickest and safest cure is to miss the next meal and have a good walk. The walk acts as a charm. One may start out looking and feeling miserable and come in cheerful and make everyone else feel so. Try this simple remedy and you will be surprised how well it acts.'

Chapter 6

BEING IN GOOD SPIRITS

WHILE Allinson had to deal with many physical ailments, he was also concerned about mental or emotional ones. And, like many holistic practitioners today, he believed they were interdependent, linked together on the most profound basis. So, symptoms that appeared to be from a wholly mental source might be improved by physical procedures. Take, for instance, that common Victorian malady, Nervousness:

'Our nerves in reality are only as so many wires loading from the brain to the muscles, organs and various parts of the body. When a person says his nerves are out of order he is not speaking correctly. His nerves have no more to do with the cause of his symptoms than the telegraph wires have to do with the messages sent over them. The brain is in reality the centre from which all movements come and to which all sensations are referred. If I prick a person's hand with a pin, he will tell me he feels the pain in his hand; but he does nothing of the kind. The pain is felt by the brain and referred to the hand. The nerve centres in the brain, which govern the movements of the hand, are at once on the alert and cause it to remove from the pin almost instantly...

'Now for our subject. Nervousness has nothing to do with the nerves. It shows the whole system is at fault and that the impure blood irritates the brain cells and produces so-called nervous symptoms. Impure blood or the presence of waste material n the blood causes other symptoms as well; and thus anger, bad temper, spleen &c are all due to improperly constituted blood.

'**Causes**: The causes of nervousness are any habits which lower the tone of the body or any foods or substances which load the system with improper materials. Too much food, too little exercise, too little fresh air and a dirty skin all tend to produce this complaint. The chief producers of it are substances which are not foods, but which are used by man in his so-called civilisation as almost necessaries of life. The most common substance which gives rise to nervous symptoms is alcohol…. It first causes unsteadiness of the muscles or paralysis of the brain cells which govern them; and if taken in sufficient quantity and for long enough, it may produce the highest of all nervous states – insanity. Next in order comes tobacco. It causes palpitation, trembling and unsteadiness very quickly. Lastly, come strong tea and coffee. To many these are nearly as bad as alcoholic liquors. Tea and coffee are poisons and cause a host of distressing symptoms.

'**Symptoms**: These vary from mere trembling to madness. Thus, after drinking tea, a person may feel more or less nervous, does not like to speak to anyone, cannot look anyone in the face and feels as if he would like to be left alone. Higher symptoms are seen when a person starts at any sudden noise, as a knock at the door. He has also sudden strange forebodings. He feels something dreadful is going to happen to himself or his friends. He worries and fidgets over little things, wonders if he has fastened all the doors at night and is not sure if he has locked the safe. Others, again, are afraid to cross the street for fear of being run over. Many will not ride in a cab or omnibus for fear the horses should fall and the idea of a railway journey is terrible. Business men will fear bankruptcy, failure or some such mishap; whilst professional men fear a decline of work, loss of social status &c. In some this feeling of hopeless ruin and misery reaches such a pitch as to occasion suicide. Other symptoms are starting of the muscles, twitching or jumping in the sleep, or even mild convulsions.

'**Cure**: Cease to do evil, learn to do well. Do not overeat. Too much food causes nervousness…. If you smoke, stop doing so, and make up your mind that you cannot afford to injure your body for a mere habit. If you take the seductive glass of liquor try to give it up; and the sooner you do so the sooner you will feel a new life never before dreamt of.'

There again, there were some ailments, too, that were dreamt up, as Allinson points out in his essay, *Hypochondria*:

'This is a peculiar disease, usually affecting the delicate or those who have insufficient work or mental stimulus. It is a condition of the system in which all kinds of symptoms, natural or abnormal, are carefully noted and worried over. A better term for this complaint would be "hypersensitiveness" that is, the brooding over ordinary things or symptoms which a person in health would not notice. They are the most difficult patients that the ordinary doctor has to deal with. The doctor suggests first one remedy and then another, recommends change of air, rest from business and such like, and then as he finds no lasting good is done, he recommends them to go to a physician. The patient, especially if he is fairly well off, goes from physician to physician, pays their fees, takes their prescriptions, and has regularly a change of treatment. No patent medicine, appliance, nor application is left untried. The patient seemingly gets a little good result from every new prescription and fresh mode of treatment, but this is only temporary, and goes off as soon as the excitement of the novelty has passed away.

'Hypochondriacs are the doctor's horror, as they come to him with a prepared list of all their symptoms; they wander off from the point, and it is only by strict and direct questioning that any consistent story can be extracted from them. They are continually trying baths, diets and other things and jumbling causes and results up together and bring the doctor a tangled web to unravel. The causes of this disease may be hereditary, delicate constitution or acquired from wrong living. As I have said before, want of sufficient occupation or of natural excitement is a great cause.

'Thus I find that most of the cases I see are among Government clerks, or those engaged in situations with but short hours, and not overmuch laborious or absorbing work to do. After these come persons of independent means, who have no need to work or occupy themselves, and who take up no study, hobby or reform with which to occupy their time. The faces of such persons show an unmistakable look of refinement, delicacy or effeminacy and they shrink from doing anything that causes prolonged thought or exertion.

'Wrong dietetic or hygienic habits play a most important part in the production of this disease. Thus overfeeding and too rich foods are one of the roots of this complaint. As a rule a larger quantity of food than the body requires is eaten, and this brings on an attack of morbidness. These people are sometimes very faddish about what they eat and drink, avoiding almost religiously certain foods and drinks.

They try and live according to the best standards they can find, yet everything they eat seems to disagree and bring on their symptoms.

'Want of exercise is another root of this condition; the sufferers do not get enough and so have plenty of time to brood over their real or fancied ailments. The signs of the complaint are numerous. Whenever a patient gives you a long list of symptoms, rambles from his subject and talks on other things that he has noticed, then you know that you have one of these cases to deal with. The commonest symptoms are matters connected with the reproductive organs, and it is on these persons that quacks play their most impudent tricks, and it is from them that they extort most money. You may know the hypochondriac by his miserableness, and he is never happy unless he can unfold a most horrible and terrible list of symptoms. He usually acts as a killjoy to the people amongst whom he goes, whilst his acquaintances and friends shun him if possible on account of the low spirits that accompany him like a shadow.

'**Cure**: The cure of this disease is slow; it must be systematic to be sure, and a firm will must be exercised over the patient. If you can get him to occupy himself in some work, either profitable or otherwise, you may assist the cure. Any work, so long as it is exciting, or that it must be done, banishes the self-consciousness. Then food must not be overlooked; its quantity and quality must be regulated. Meat or animal food must be eaten very sparingly, better still if your patient will consent to abstain from it altogether, and the quantity of food must also be regulated. Simple food eaten to excess will give rise to the symptoms; you must try and find out the exact quantity which suits the patient, without causing morbid feelings. When this amount is found out, then your patient must rigidly adhere to it. Much sugar, jam, cream, rich foods, greasy foods, artificial or made dishes are all bad; plainly cooked food, and not in large portions, is the best. If alcoholic drinks and tobacco are taken, they must be discontinued. Daily, regular and systematic exercise of any or all kinds is most valuable and will cure an attack of this disease more rapidly than anything else. Fresh air must not be despised; continually breathing it aids cure. Bathing, especially the cold bath, is a useful remedy; daily tepid, or cold bathing and swimming are good. Drugs of all kinds are usually harmful, and even if harmless, they raise false expectations. Travel, change of scene or excitement of any kind is good. The means of cure are varied and the improvement slow, but following the directions given on the above lines gives the most success.'

PART THREE: HYGIENIC LIVING

Chapter 1

ALLINSON'S LONG WALK

N O ONE could ever accuse Allinson of not practising what he preached. In 1891, he undertook a challenge to prove that a vegetarian diet could provide all the strength that might be needed by anyone, whatever he or she might be doing. 'Friends often told him such a diet was, no doubt, good for mental work and strain, but not for physical exertion. To prove the fallacy of these people, he quietly undertook to walk this distance, and at the end of the journey convince them of their error,' said a newspaper account of his efforts. In true Allinsonian fashion, he walked from Edinburgh to London. This is the account given in the press:

'Near the end of August 1891 he sailed to Edinburgh, stayed a day with some friends, and then began his walk. On Saturday August 29, he and a companion left the General Post Office, Edinburgh at 11.15am, and walked 28 miles to Crosslee; on Sunday he got to Burnside Ewes, which is 37 miles from Crosslee; on Tuesday he arrived at Carlisle, 27 1/2 miles from Burnside Ewes. From Carlisle he walked to Shap in one day, a distance of 29 miles; next day he walked to Carnforth, a distance of 31 1/2 miles; next day brought him to Preston, 28 1/2 miles from his last resting place.

'From Preston he walked to Burnley, a distance of 20^1/$_2$ miles; next day he proceeded to Oldham, a distance of 24 miles; from Oldham he waled 26^1/$_2$ miles into Buxton. The distance from Buxton to Belper is 31 miles, and this done in a day; next day he walked from Belper to Leicester, a distance of 35 miles. After leaving Leicester he walked 16 miles for Market Harborough, and stopped there at night as he could not get a bed at any of the places a few miles ahead. Leaving Market Harborough, he walked that day to Newport Pagnell, a distance of 32 miles. From Newport Pagnell to Welwyn is a distance of 35 miles, which as done in one day; lastly, on Saturday, Sept 12, he finished his walk from Welwyn to London, a distance of 25 miles.

'He did not walk the nearest, nor the least hilly way, but so arranged that he called in some of his friends on the way. He walked for fifteen consecutive days, on an average of nearly 28 miles a day. Dr Allinson's companion only accomplished 50 miles on foot, then his feet became so blistered that he had to rest a day, and finish the rest on his bicycle. This gentleman accompanied Dr Allinson all the way, rode ahead and had meals ready, and chose the quarters for the night. The distances given do not always represent the distances travelled, as he was misdirected sometimes, or got out of his road, and so walked more than necessary.

'The weather was not often favourable; the third, fourth and ninth days were very wet, and had to be walked with an open umbrella, and a wind blowing almost dead against him. Three times he was wet through, twice his clothes dried on him, but once he had put on the suit of the landlord of the hotel where he put up for the night, whilst his own dried. The wind was against him all the way, and when it blew and rained together it made progression difficult. The last four or five days the sun shone fiercely on him, and made him freely perspire. His meals were usually two a day; at first he had a good breakfast, and then no more food until he finished his day's walk, then his second meal, a rest of a few hours, and to bed. The day he walked from Carlisle to Shap, which is 29 miles, he walked the whole distance without a stop and without taking food and drink until he had finished, and, as it was both windy and wet, he had a rough time of it, for the road lies on the top of the hills all the way, and is not much protected by trees.

'His luggage at first consisted of a dust coat and some papers, but after three days the coat was sent home by Parcel-post, and his cyclist friend carried the papers; then his luggage consisted of an umbrella, a fairly heavy roadbook, and some money. His dress consisted of a soft cap which was mostly carried in his pocket, a shooting jacket, in which were extra pockets to contain watch, comb, toothbrush and a few useful odds and ends; instead of trousers he wore breeches; long stockings covered his legs; he wore ordinarily strong boots, with some large nails driven in the soles; a Net of Health vest was worn next the skin, over this a flannel cricketing shirt, but no waistcoat.

'He had some little difficulty with his food and, not knowing the road, had to put up where he could get a bed; one night he slept at the house of a farm labourer, and one night, after wandering about for two hours, he was received into the house of a gentleman farmer – this at nearly eleven at night, no tavern within ten miles of him. Yet, in spite of all these disadvantages, he has accomplished his walk, and done a fair average for a man who is engaged in professional work all day. His walk shows what can be done without beef or beer – also that Dr Allinson is not without perseverance, which is so characteristic of our English race.

Chapter 2

ALLINSON'S STAGES OF LIFE

ALLINSON believed hygienic living should be practised throughout life and had advice for every stage. Victorian living had very high rates of infant mortality, most notably in cities, and he thought that children and babies would have a better chance of health by changing their diet and giving them the chance to take plenty of fresh air and exercise. *Management of Infancy* was his first essay in his first collection – perhaps an indication of the importance he attached to getting the first years right:

'Half the children born alive never reach the age of five years. That a great many of these premature deaths are avoidable may be judged from the fact that in some country districts there have been no deaths of children for many years... .

'When a child is born the first thing to do is to wrap it up in a piece of flannel until the mother is made comfortable. Then the child should be washed in warm water with some very bland soap, dried carefully and not clothed as children are usually in all kinds of wraps and constraints, but in some things which allow of perfect freedom of the limbs, without tightness anywhere. The custom of putting bands round babies and dressing them up in costly clothes is a sop thrown to the goddess fashion and is positively injurious... .

'There is much ignorance with regard to the food baby should be given until the mother's milk comes. The common plan of giving gruel, butter and sugar, sugar and water &c is bad. The natural plan is to put baby to its mother's breast a few hours after birth... . This plan is beneficial to both mother and child. It prevents many troubles to the mother. The first milk is always rich in fat and when baby draws this into its stomach it acts as a natural purgative and moves the bowels... .

If the mother will take wheatmeal gruel and brown bread with fruits and vegetables after baby's birth for her food, she will require no purgatives on the third or any other day. I write this plainly because when in general practice I saw much ill-health and suffering result from ignorance of such things. The less medicines at these as at other times the better.

'All mothers should suckle their children if possible. The reason is that the mother's milk is most natural for her baby and as the baby grows, the milk of the mother gradually changes and so the baby goes through natural stages in the proper order… When a baby is given the breast it knows how much to take and stops when it feels satisfied. Not so with artificial food, which may be made sweet and so baby takes more than is good for it. The results of over feeding are fretfulness, crossness, irritability, sleeplessness and other symptoms which are characteristic of a so-called bad-tempered child. If full grown persons were fed too often, no matter however simple the food, they would soon be bad tempered and their wives would vote them not fit to live with, yet we overfeed our babies and then expect them to be models of goodness…. Many mothers imagine that they will not have milk enough to feed a baby unless they drink stout, porter, beer or some such filthy stuff. I am sorry to say they are often encouraged in this delusion by their family doctor and the nurse….

'Infants must not be given any solid food until they cut at least two teeth…. The first solid food a child has must be a proper food and one capable of sustaining baby and supplying its organs with what they want. Such food in this country is the grain of wheat, oats or barley, in other words a child's first food should be either fine wheatmeal or oatmeal or barley-meal. I am very particular about the first food supplied to children, as a great deal of future misery or happiness depends on the food given during the first few years of life…. When children are fed on white bread sop, on rusks, on tops and bottoms and especially if fed on arrowroot, sago &c, they do not get enough bone-forming materials in their blood and become rickety; that is, their bones bend and they become bow-legged, pigeon chested &c. They may suffer from constipation and other ailments as well and then grow up delicate, nervous and miserable people, instead of good, strong, lusty men and women. Children fed on wholemeal bread are more likely to become tall in stature than those fed on white bread... .

'After a child is two years old and if healthy and strong, he may be allowed vegetables and a little plain pudding at dinner. Split peas, haricot beans, lentils, cheese, eggs, fish, flesh or fowl should not be given to children before they are two years of age. After that age, an egg two or three times a week may be allowed at dinner. Bacon, pork, ham, veal, cod liver oil, Yorkshire and suet puddings, Norfolk and Christmas puddings &c should not be given. Pastry and cakes, also sweets and nuts should not be allowed under two years and afterwards only sparingly... .

'Babies should have two baths daily, a lukewarm one in the morning and a warmer one at night. These should be continued until the child is about eighteen months old, then it may have a bath with the chill off every morning and its hands and face sponged two or three times a day... . Bathing has a double action, first that of keeping the millions of skin pores open and so allowing waste material to easily escape from the body. Secondly, it acts as a tonic, by exposing the naked skin to the cold air. This exposure tempers or hardens the skin, tones the system and so makes them less liable to colds. In connection with bathing, if the sun is shining, it will do baby good to expose the naked body to its warm rays for a little time... .

'The inestimable importance of fresh air to babies is not sufficiently known... . Its crib, cot or cradle must not be surrounded with curtains keeping out the fresh air... . The bedroom in which baby sleeps should have the window open a little and the room in which it is kept during the day should also have the window open a little. After baby is 14 days old it may go out every day, or even twice a day. The best time to take a child out is when the sun is shining, but it should be sent out every day unless the weather is wet or snowy. Windy weather does not hurt the child, but puts colour on its cheeks. I appeal to all mothers if this fact I name is not true, "children become less cross and irritable the moment they go out, and in most cases they soon fall asleep"... .

'A baby should be taken out in a perambulator daily and of perambulators the best kind is that in which baby can lie at full length. At home baby may be laid on the bed on his back and allowed to throw his arms and legs about. As he gets older he may be put on the floor and allowed to crawl about. Never force a child to walk, nor fret because he does not walk as soon as some other child does… when a child can once walk you must expect him to go everywhere and be in every kind of mischief. He is not content with walking, but must climb also, as the arm muscles want exercise as well as those of the leg. Sensible parents will provide some simple apparatus for their offspring to indulge in climbing without danger. Children will not exercise too much. When they are tired they will stop or will come indoors and fall asleep until rested. It is a mistake to curb children and be afraid of letting them tire themselves. It is also a mistake to make them be still. Every house should have space for them where they can romp and play to their heart's content; and when friends visit one another, the children of both should be let loose in the garden or nursery whilst the older folks enjoy a social talk… .

'Children have really an aversion to clothes, as we know by the fact that they always pull them off when they can… . The fact that many mothers will not let their children go out to play without they wear an overcoat and a muffler is deplorable. The muffled-up child cannot exercise properly, it soon perspires, is easily fatigued and quickly takes cold. Had the child gone out in ordinary clothing, it would have been able to play about freely, the perspiration would escape easily and the child would be pounds better for the exercise… .

'Babies must never be given drugs or medicines, as they are more readily killed by such things than are adults. So called soothing, cooling and teething powders have hurried thousands to an early grave. Medicines and powders given by drug doctors are even more harmful and many a sorrowing mother would now have her baby to comfort her had she thrown the medicines down the drain instead of giving them to her tender babe. The same applies to brandy and wine. I never use medicines or intoxicants (so called stimulants) in my practice and rarely lose a child.'

Allinson gave advice on the rearing of older children in a later essay, *The Management of Children*. He was particularly keen on fresh air and exercise, recommending, 'The longer children are out in the open air the better for them. Let them be out in all weathers; wind will give colour to their cheeks, the sun will tan them and the rain will not harm them. Frost makes them run about to keep warm and the cold weather invigorates them. Present your boys with barrows, spades, balls, hoops and the implements of rational games. Give the girls balls, hoops and a skipping rope, also a battledoor and shuttlecock. Let the children run about and be as noisy as ever they like; if you have some place for them separate from yourselves, turn them into it and let them enjoy themselves to their hearts' content. At the seaside let them paddle, wade or bathe and be without shoes and stockings all day long if they choose. If in the country, let them be out all day like country children. Very little learning should be allowed before six; the rudiments of the three R's as they are called may be taught but never keep your children more than an hour or two each day at their studies.'

A long, long life

Allinson believed that everyone could – if they tailored their way of life according to his advice – live to 70. Given that the average life expectancy of the time was just 43, this was an extraordinary claim. In an essay, *Longevity*, he sets out his case:

'The question of man's age is one simply of calculation based on certain lines. Most animals live six times the period they take in coming to puberty, some say to maturity. Man attains puberty about the age of fifteen; and if we multiply this by six, we get ninety years as being man's proper age at the time of death. If we reckon by maturity, we get a longer period. Man comes to maturity from twenty to twenty-five years; and if we take the lower number for calculation and multiply by six as before, we get a hundred and twenty years as man's natural age at death... .

'If a man is regular in his habits, temperate in food and drink, has some regular occupation and can attain philosophic calmness to take the world as he finds it, then he may live out his allotted time. But if he is irregular in his habits, intemperate in food and drink, if he smokes, breathes vitiated or poisoned air and takes no care of himself, then he will die before his natural time... . If we respect our persons in their physical conditions these organs will last out their time, but if we do otherwise the will fail and bring the body to premature dissolution. I can only finish with an almost unknown quotation:"He who dies under seventy is guilty of physical suicide."

Allinson himself was to die at sixty. In *How Persons Have Lived 100*

Years, he relates the story of a remarkable man. 'One of the oldest men whose record we have is that of "Old Jenkins", who lived to 169. He lived in the country as a farmer, worked regularly on his land and attended to his cattle all the year round. In those days the food of the people would consist mainly of barley bread, oatmeal, milk, fruits and a few green vegetables. Prepared foods, foods from abroad and the hundred and one delicacies we have nowadays were unheard of by him. Pepper, mustard, condiments, spices, sugar, pickles and other like things were unknown to him as would be grapes, oranges, bananas, lemons &c. His bread would be made from barley meal and raised with a piece of old leaven and not with barm or yeast. His drinks would be water, milk and water, buttermilk and a kind of light ale, very little stronger than ordinary ginger beer. Tea, coffee and cocoa or almost any hot drink would be little used by him. The meals of people at the time he lived were at six, eleven and four and to bed at eight. Tobacco was almost unknown or the use of it had not extended to his neighbourhood. His house would be a shelter for him and not airtight; the windows had no glass in them, but would be open all day and closed at night with a shutter, being in reality wind-doors. The house would be one storey, the chimney being wide and capacious, acted as a good ventilator. Lamps and gas were unknown, his candle would be of tallow and rush and not many of them, as early retiring to rest was the rule. Baths were unknown and he probably never had one, or only an occasional summer one. There were no daily posts, morning and evening papers never excited him, nor telegrams troubled him. Trains and such things were unknown. He rarely stirred far from his native place; his village was his world.... .

'Monks of some orders live long. The Trappists who live on vegetarian diet, who never use tobacco and rarely wine, who work hard all day in the fields, retire early and get up early are noted for their long lives. Their clothes are simplicity itself; a habit fastened round the waist with a rope girdle and sandals for the feet. They never wash as they ought to do. Yet they are seldom ill and rarely die before eighty. Hermits in the same way, fare poorly, are simply clad and badly housed; yet they live long. The simple food and habits of the Quakers and Shakers are also conducive to long life.

'**Moral**: Live simply; the simpler your food and the nearer it is to the state obtained from our fields and gardens, the longer you will live. Exercise daily, get all the pure air you can and avoid artificiality as much as possible. Tea, coffee, tobacco, stimulants, spices and condiments, hot things and tasty dishes, must be avoided as they bring on disease and shorten life.'

Life and Pleasure

At times, Allinson sounds somewhat restrictive in his rules for hygienic living but then he also recommends many simple pleasures as a means of improving health. He was, for instance, very keen on promoting the idea of holidays. In the Twenty-First Century, when everyone takes multiple holidays, this may seem a strange idea. However, in the Nineteenth Century, very few people took holidays at all, working long hours in often dark and insanitary buildings – Allinson did not approve at all:

'Recreation,' he declared in an essay in his first collection, *Holidays*, 'really means a change of scene or of occupation; thus a hard working mechanic would be recreating himself if he laid on a sandy beach all day, looked up at the sky and tried to solve some of the many problems that every day trouble him. The ardent student should relax himself by throwing aside his books and having a spell of hard physical work or by walking, rowing, tricycling &c. The country person enjoys a run into a busy town to see its wonders; whilst the seaside dweller should go away to hills or mountains. By this means we get not only a change of occupation but also a change of scene and our minds become renovated as well as our bodies... .

'The best time of year for an enjoyable holiday is the summer or early autumn. The country is then looking its best, the days are fine and long, fruit is ripe, the scent of flowers fills the air and all nature is gay and compels one's admiration. The next question is, where shall we go? Town dwellers who have friends and relatives in the country should go there, especially if there are children and not too much spare cash. Those without country friends should go to some country farm-house where the children can have plenty of fresh milk, fruit and vegetables and can be out in the open air all day long, dirty themselves as much as they please and put on their old clothes and tear them without being scolded. This is the true pleasure of children. At the same time as the children are running wild and getting the last wear out of their old clothes, their parents may visit all the ruins, remarkable churches and old curiosities in the neighbourhood – and there are very few places that have not some remarkable histories or associations. Let the young man without wife or encumbrances have a walking or tricycling tour or a stay at the seaside with its morning bath and the afternoon walk or its row… .You will gain an immense reserve of vital force and strength and return to your customary work like giants refreshed.'

In fact, Allinson clearly had a vision of what we would now call the work-life balance. In *Work and Overwork*, one of his fourth collection essays, he puts forward some very modern views:

'The desire to establish a good business or to make provision for one's old age or one's family is a wise determination but if we try to do this too quickly we may defeat our own ends… .We often hear of, or may personally know, some who work early and late and deny themselves rightful rest or relaxation that they may get together a good business connection and when they have done so and are hoping to reap the reward of their self-sacrificing labours, then disease, due to the violation of the laws of life cuts them off in what should be the very prime of their days… . Every business man should take two hours' exercise in the open air daily. No man should excuse himself and say he has no time; he must make time or his health will fail and his business necessarily suffer… .Those who work hard with the brain all day must rest at night from their work and use their muscles instead before they sleep. Debility of all kinds, low spirits, insanity and consumption often attack those who work at the desk early and late and who neglect exercise.'

In *Summer Living*, from the first collection of essays, he wholeheartedly endorses the weekend away. 'To those who can afford it, I should say, run away from Saturday to Monday, as it will do you a world of good and the money you spend in or on your trips will be saved in doctors' bills.' Of course, the summer lent itself to many of the activities Allinson favoured both for health and pleasure. 'Summer is the time,' he advised, 'when we should acquire a stock of vitality so that we may have a reserve fund should such ever be needed.'

He recommends light foods. 'Salads are cooling on account of the water and mild acids they contain,' he says. 'Those who desire clear complexions cannot do better than eat freely of salads as they are among the best blood purifiers known.... Ripe fruit of all kinds can be eaten freely. Let each kind be eaten as it comes in season and great benefit will result.'

He also suggests making as much use as possible of the fine weather. 'From the middle or the end of May bathing may be commenced, in the sea or in fresh water. Two or three baths a week should be taken if possible, whilst those who have the time and opportunity may take one daily. A daily swim is useful in many ways. It acts as a tonic to the system generally, while the action of the sun and air on the naked skin is very invigorating. Even the most delicate may begin to have a sponge down in the morning. Those whose lives are chiefly spent in offices should get up early and have a swim before breakfast. It will keep them fresh all day.

'The bedroom windows should be kept wide open; nothing calms one so much as the cool night air...Exercise must be taken systematically, the long days allowing persons to be up early and out late, before and after office hours. Young folks must now polish up their "wheel machines" and take daily runs or they may row on the river.... .

'My young lady readers cannot do better than join a lawn tennis club and practise daily or they may get their brother or someone else's brother to take them for a run on a social or tandem tricycle. A word in season as to clothing. Wear light things. Those who dare should now wear straw hats and light-coloured clothes, and then they may be in comfort, whilst their more unfortunate friends are sweltering in uncomfortable black coats and nonsensical tall hats.'

Chapter 3

THE SHAPE OF THINGS TO COME

HIS RECOMMENDATIONS on clothing for young ladies did not end with advice about outer-garments, however. In *Stays and their Subsitutes*, he offers advice that would at the time have been quite shocking, not just in its frank discussion of women's undergarments and bodies, but in the suggestion that by taking such matters into their own hands, they were insisting on freedom from and even equality with men:

'The habit of wearing stays or corsets is one dating from the dark ages... . In bygone days they were often made of iron, covered with fine leather and forcibly compressed the waist and bust of their unfortunate wearers so that they could scarcely breathe. With an increased knowledge of ourselves has come a revolution in dress and corsets have undergone a reform like everything else. Many of our sensible women nowadays do not wear them and their number increases daily. Women are becoming more educated and free and are not such slaves to fashion as in former years; one result of this is the partial abandonment of these injurious articles of attire.

'Stays or corsets may be defined as articles of dress which compress the contents of the chest and stomach; they are worn mostly by ladies, also by a few men. The reasons given for wearing them are that they are supposed to keep the middle part of the body neat looking... Let us take a common sense view and bring facts to bear on the subject. It has been shown that ladies who wear corsets cannot breathe so freely as those who do not; those who have them on lose a third of their breathing space... . On the abdominal organs the effect of stays is well marked; the liver is compressed and often shows a deep dent

or line on post mortem examinations. Its functions are interfered with...
.The stomach is contracted.... and indigestion is a result. Corsets force
the bowels themselves downwards and do not allow them to act with
proper freedom. This compression of the abdominal contents means
pressure on the large vein returning blood from the legs to the heart;
the results are varicose veins of the legs, piles and even ulcers of the
legs.... The greatest evil of all is to the womb and reproductive organs;
these are forced out of their natural position and cause an immense
number of diseases peculiar to women. It can be safely said that about
three-quarters of the womb troubles from which women suffer are due
to corset wearing. The discomfort, uneasiness and poor health caused by
such displacements are incalculable and they support a large army of
specialist doctors who treat diseases of women only. These, instead of
recommending rational living and clothing, do all kinds of useless and
often injurious operations and expose women to all the horrors of
special appliances, pessaries &c and repeated examinations. Life is a
burden to many women merely on account of these appliances.

'During pregnancy corsets are very harmful and may prevent the
proper growth of the child, its imperfect development or premature
confinement.... We will now enquire into the reasons why stays are
worn. The first is because it is the fashion to do so, and some women
would rather be out of the world than out of the fashion.... The next
is that ladies think corsets make them look neat and trim and not like
sacks of flour; but ladies who wear corsets have an angular look that
is anything but artistic; in fact, all our well known artists paint from the
nude so that they may portray the graceful curves of the natural figure.

'To artistic minds small waists are ugly, as they spoil the figure and
disturb the natural proportions. Let sensible young men be warned,
and make it one of the conditions in the future wife that she be
stayless; if she "draws in" very much, look out for a cheerless house and
a wife who prefers fashion and frivolity rather than the joys and
comforts of a home.... I am pleased to say that Mrs Allinson had given
up wearing stays before I knew her.... [and she] is neater about the
waist than most women and the lines of her figure are natural and
graceful, yet she wears no corsets.

Some say stays prevent their becoming too stout. A simpler way to
keep slim is not to overeat and to take more exercise.'

Fat is a Victorian issue

Incredibly, that, too, was regarded as an unusual view in the Nineteenth Century. But Allinson went further – he believed obesity was a threat to health, an unheard of notion at the time:

'Obesity, corpulence, stoutness, fatness, embonpoint and full bodiedness are the names usually given to that state of the body in which there is superfluous bulk. This flesh is not muscle and is not a sign of health, but simply so much fat or waste matter. I consider that if we allow to adults two pounds to the inch in height, we give a fair average, that is a person of 5ft 6in in height, is not stout if not above 9st 6lbs in weight. This is a rough rule and holds good from eighteen years of age to about sixty years... . Obesity is a disease and like every other disease injures the system.

'**Causes**: The causes are many but they may be summed up in one sentence, viz, the taking of more food than the system can use. The amount will vary; thus a cripple and a hard-working man should not eat the same amount of food; nor should a clerk or one leading an indoor life, eat as much as one doing hard work. The great cause of obesity is over-feeding; next to this comes want of exercise; thirdly, the retention of waste matter in the system... .

'Many people are of the opinion that the more food men or women eat the better they must be. This is a delusion; every person requires a certain amount of food for the wear and tear of the body and the proper performance of the bodily functions, and more than is required for this is harmful. It does harm because force is used up in absorbing the excess of food and again in getting rid of it. Every person must find out the exact amount necessary for himself; if he eats only three meals a day of plain food, stops at the first feeling of satisfaction, and does not force himself to eat when not hungry, he cannot go far wrong. If he still finds that he is increasing in weight above the average I have given, then he should cut down the quantity.

'The nature of the food also may cause obesity. Thus: all the starchy, sugary, oily and fatty foods cause stoutness. The starchy foods are potatoes, rice, sago, tapioca, macaroni, hominy, cornflour &c. The sugary foods are the dried fruits, carrots and artificial sugars. The oily and fatty foods are cream, butter, cheese some fishes, fat fowls and fat meats. The vegetable fat foods are olives and nuts.

'When food is not burnt up by exercise, fatness results. Exercise burns up excess of food by consuming it in the form of work; exercise also carries more oxygen into the system and this burns up waste. Men who are active and busy with their bodies rarely get stout; thus one rarely ever sees a fat soldier, sailor or anyone daily engaged in active duty. But porters, policemen, watchmen and others who lead a life of not too active a nature soon put on flesh. Persons who lead a sedentary life are stouter than those who do not... .

'The last cause of obesity is the result of waste matter being left in the body. Alcohol in the form of beer, wines or spirits causes retention of waste in the system and so gives rise to obesity. Alcohol prevents the blood from freely carrying oxygen into the system, waste of all sorts is retained and obesity results. This is the worst kind of stoutness, common amongst brewers' men and drinkers of all sorts; it is bloatedness and diseasedness. Tobacco is another cause of stoutness, as it slows the heart's action, the blood does not get sufficiently purified and the waste left in the system causes an increase in weight... .

'**Results**: Stoutness causes an increased weight of the body; this makes it more difficult to get about. In races men handicap horses by making them carry extra weight, but human beings handicap themselves when there is no necessity, consequently they do not win so many of life's prizes as they might and they certainly do not get the best one of all, viz, health. Stoutness makes locomotion more difficult and so helps to increase itself. The mass of fat also injures other organs, especially the heart, for if an ounce of fat is deposited on that organ it has to be lifted every time the heart beats. We also find stout persons subject to bronchitis and breathlessness on exertion. They cannot go uphill, upstairs or anywhere without being out of breath. In disease they have not the stamina of thinner persons; they are rarely long lived and may die from diabetes, apoplexy, syncope, &c.

'**Cure**: The cure is difficult, as we have to carry it out ourselves. In the first place I must warn my readers against remedies of all sorts, such as strong acids, anti-fat remedies and such like. The cure is a careful diet and regular exercise, with the avoidance of alcoholic stimulants and bad air. Here I must warn my readers against the "Banting Cure" and the hot water and meat dietary cures. They are starvation cures of the worst kind. The Banting cure is to eat chiefly of meat, whilst the other in addition to drink freely of warm or hot water. The Banting cure pulls down the weight and loads the system with waste; whilst the Salisbury Cure as it is called, starves the patients and ruins the stomach by the quantity of hot water taken. I have seen some very bad cases of stomach disease produced by this meat and hot water cure.'

So it appears that the Victorians had their own version of the Atkins diet. While Allinson didn't approve of faddy diets he did believe that fasting was beneficial from time to time:

'So usual is it for persons to indulge too freely in food, that religion has stepped in and given her sanction to abstinence and made it a virtue. All great religions have organised fast days which are beneficial to the health if people will observe them. Looked at from a purely medical point of view, we find some very interesting and instructive results take place on lessening the quantity of food eaten. We find first that the body loses nearly all its fat; this is the first tissue that is absorbed, being waste that the body cannot use… . The spleen is the next organ that loses weight; an enlarged spleen is as dangerous as an enlarged liver and as incurable. The liver follows by lessening in size and after a fast of some days loses a good deal of its waste matters. Those who are troubled with congestion of the liver, pain in the right shoulder or between the shoulders and who feel heavy, dull and without energy, will do well to lessen the quantity of their food and so unload this organ. A starve for one day will cure or cut short a bilious attack very quickly. The muscles do not lose much weight from fasting, so that although a person feels weak from going without food, he is not really much weaker unless he fasts to excess. The blood loses about a fifth of its nourishment from fasting; this is often very useful. To clear the blood, to lessen congestion in the head, and to bring down the pulse, a starve is the best thing. It requires self-control to submit to this, but the results are good and no diseases follow as they do when poisonous drugs are taken… .

'The stout, the plethoric or full blooded or those who suffer from the effects of overfeeding, as the bilious and dyspeptic, will find it useful to go without a meal, and instead take only a drink of water or a cup of gruel. Josh Billings said, "A doctor should be a gentleman who tells you to exercise more and eat less." If people would apply this advice in their choice of doctors what a number of doctors would have to turn bankrupt or exercise their ingenuity in other ways. A common-sense old friend one day told me that he often did me out of a fee by taking a long walk and going without a meal, whenever he felt bilious or out of sorts. A man who lived to be 180 years old attributed his long life to the fact that he only ate one meal a day, took all his food cold and fasted the first and fifteenth of every month.... To miss a meal occasionally does one more good than a feast.'

Chapter 4

PURE WATER AND SUNSHINE

WHILE Allinson recommended missing the occasional meal, one of the things he believed you could not do without was pure water. And the emphasis was very much on its purity, defined by him in such a way that bottlers of mineral water may find uncomfortable reading. In an essay entitled *Pure Water* from his fifth and final collection of essays, he lays out his case:

'Water in itself is not a food, but yet life cannot go on without it; it is the channel by which foods are absorbed into the system and waste matters are dissolved and removed. Three-fourths of the weight of the human body consists of water; thus if a man weigh 100lbs, 25lbs of solid parts are all that will remain when all the fluid has been driven off. The food we eat must contain three-quarters water or that equivalent must be taken with dry food, otherwise we experience thirst... .

'The chief use of water being to act as a solvent, it follows that the purer the water the better will it fulfil its functions. Water varies very much in its composition; rain water gathered in the country some distance from a town is the purest. It is composed of almost pure water and if it is caught from a clean roof and stored in clean receptacles it is the perfection of what water ought to be.'

In *Light*, he argues that sunshine and the open air gave another free, yet inestimable, benefit to health. 'Who does not know,' he asks, 'the good influence of a bright day on the mind and temper? There are some people so constituted that their very spirits depend in a great measure on the weather. Is it bright and cheerful, they are well; but is it dull and dark, they become depressed and dispirited. As it is with these peculiarly constituted ones so is it more or less with all of us. A bright day makes us feel well and a dull one more or less miserable. If we will glance around us we may see some cause for all this. Looking first at plants we find that those grown in dark cellars or gloomy places are always pale and blanched; whilst in rooms, that side of the plant which is next the light has always the most leaves on and all the branches grow towards the light. Plants brought up in plenty of light thrive well and cheer us by their beauty.

'Among the inferior animals we find light necessary for growth and development. It is said that tadpoles will never become frogs if they are kept always in the dark. Animals in a state of nature bask in the sun and revel in its life-giving rays; human beings greatly improve by being much in its light; while those brought up in cellars or dark rooms are pale, sickly looking, languid and without energy. Who does not envy the brown, sturdy gypsy child; and who is not proud of his brown sun-burnt face after a holiday? A person with a good colour is said to look well. Absence of light must often mean an absence of air; absence of both is soon followed by disease. If we compare the mortality of the sunny and the shady sides of a street we find that most deaths occur on the dark side. In Italy the rent of rooms is higher in some of the towns as you ascend, for as you are elevated you get more light and sunshine. The Italians have a saying, "Where the sun does not enter, the doctor does."

'Many people are afraid of the sun and try to exclude it from their rooms by blinds and curtains. Could I but banish all blinds and curtains and light obstructors I would. If persons are afraid of the sun spoiling their carpets, let them put some druggeting over them or else buy such carpets as will not fade. If the sun makes their rooms hot, well and good, they can then open their windows and cool their rooms by fresh air. Knowing the value of light and its influence on the body I never sleep with my blinds down, nor will I allow my blinds to be pulled down when the hot afternoon sun is shining into my room. I also walk by preference in the sun and not in the shade, for I am not afraid of sunstroke, since I live correctly.'

Chapter 5

VICTORIAN SELF-IMPROVEMENT

THE NINETEENTH Century was a time when the masses in the towns and cities made great strides in 'improving themselves'. This often took the form of attending courses at night schools and working mens' colleges. Allinson believed it could be applied to a whole variety of matters including health and even appearance. He therefore wrote a serious of 'how to' essays in his third volume, the first one, not surprisingly devoted to his favourite subject.

How to Eat Properly

'Good results depend on little things and it is trifles which make life easy or unpleasant. These axioms apply equally to bodily conditions; it is on the doing of little things properly that our health depends. This is specially true with regard to eating. Chew your food well, eat it slowly and you have solved half the cure of dyspepsia, leanness &c. Swedenborg relates that once, when he was eating his breakfast, Christ appeared to him in one corner of the room, said, "Eat slowly" and then gradually disappeared. Mr Gladstone gave out a few years ago that he allowed from thirty-two to thirty-six bites to all the solid food he ate. These examples show us the regard that great men pay to little things, as on them great results depend.

'Adults with a full set of teeth have thirty-two in the mouth. Those who have lost the natural ones cannot do better than get a good artificial set, they repay the money spent… . Well chewing the food is good in at least four ways. First, the food is thoroughly minced and so the gastric and various intestinal juices can extract the nourishment from it. Secondly, the act of chewing forces saliva from the various glands and so enables what we eat to be swallowed more readily.

Thirdly, the saliva changes starch into sugar, which is then absorbed from the stomach and we get a feeling of satisfaction at the proper time. Lastly, by eating slowly we know when we are satisfied better than if we almost shovel our food down. Sloppy foods are apt to be swallowed too hurriedly but if taken with bread we eat them more leisurely. The practice of eating hard food at every meal is good, as this enables us to chew the softer foods with the harder ones. For this reason brown bread should be eaten at every meal and with every dish. Bread should be eaten with soup, porridge and pudding; in fact, with every dish for in chewing the bread we chew the other food as well. The bread also brings out the flavour of most foods by contrast. I believe one German definition of a gentleman is "a person who eats bread at every meal."

'Time must be allowed for our meals. I spend about two hours a day over my three meals. I begrudge the time and wish I could open a door in my stomach and push the food in. But as I cannot, I submit to Nature's decree and eat slowly. From twenty to thirty minutes should be spent over breakfast and tea and from thirty to forty-five over dinner.... To eat properly we must not drink during the meal.... Drink comes best at the end of a meal; it must not be hot and should be held in the mouth half a minute before being swallowed.... .

Those persons who bolt their food or swallow it rapidly often become very thin in the body, but more especially thin in the face and their tempers are not always angelic. The typical Yankee is thin faced in a great measure because he swallows his meals in the smallest possible amount of time. In America a large amount of dyspepsia and its attendant evils result from this habit.'

How to keep warm

Allinson believed hygienic living should be applied to all practical areas of everyday life. He was particularly concerned about that combination of common Victorian practices – overdressing, stuffy rooms, invalids being cosseted under blankets on the chaise longue and lack of exercise due to a lot of time being spent by just about everyone hunched over a fire. Allinson was appalled by all of this and took a diametrically opposite view – and a decidedly bracing one – when it came to keeping warm and cultivating rude good health:

'Being cold,' he opined, 'is not injurious, especially if one can get warm afterwards; while moderate exposure to cold is good, as it tones up the body, and exercises that set of nerves which regulates its heat. We have nerves whose function is to keep the body always at one heat; exposure to cold air exercises these and keeps them in good order, so that if subjected to a sudden chill these nerves are equal to the occasion and prevent internal congestions which would otherwise follow. All persons should accustom their skins to exposure by a daily air bath and be in a nude condition for at least a quarter of an hour out of the twenty-four, usually in the morning whilst washing. After washing the hands, face and neck, the body should be rubbed all over with a rough dry towel and if the fingers feel cold, they may be rubbed on the arms, body and legs until warm, just before dressing. Many imagine that as the cold weather comes on they must take more fatty and greasy foods. This is a mistake, only a slightly larger quantity of our everyday food is required.

'**How to get warm** – 1st, breathe pure air and breathe deeply; the pure air burns up the carbonaceous matter in our systems and heat is thereby produced, which is then carried to all parts of the body by the blood circulating through them. Taking long, slow and deep breaths is like blowing a fire and warms us readily by increasing oxidation of combustible matters. The bad air of a hot room warms up temporarily, but not permanently and makes us more liable to feel the cold when we go out. 2ndly, exercise freely; do it steadily and the system will soon glow with heat. Walk or run. If the feet are cold, stamp them; if the hands are cold shake and rub them. If you cannot get out of doors, go through a few simple indoor gymnastic exercises. Move all the limbs in a regular way; warm blood will soon be sent to them and all over the body as well at a quick rate. Here is a recipe for making one log of wood keep you warm all winter: Take it to the top room of the house and throw it out of the window, fetch it up, throw it out again, fetch it up again and continue until warm. Repeat as often as necessary; the log is not worn out in one winter.

'One should only take warm drinks after coming in cold and intending to remain at home, for these warm the surface by dilating the blood vessels and if we go out in the cold whilst these are dilated, we may get a chill. Warming ourselves by the fire is not good and should be practised as little as possible. Feeble constitutions must be made stronger by careful living, regular exercise and avoidance of tea, coffee, tobacco and alcohol. Those whose lungs are diseased must breathe all the pure air possible; no medicine is equal to this. Overcoats should only be worn if travelling, or if standing about, but never whilst taking exercise. Instead of closely woven flannel undergarments, loosely woven garments of cotton, wool, silk or a combination of these should be worn next the skin. These retain a layer of warm air next to the skin and do not keep it hot and moist as flannel does. To have warm feet in bed, a pair of specially knit lambswool socks may be worn at night. Those who take a walk just before going to bed, rarely suffer from cold feet during the night, their bedrooms do not seem chilly and the sheets do not strike cold. There is not any objection to a little fire in a bedroom at night if the window be kept open at least two inches.'

How to grow tall

However, Allinson did not advise only on everyday matters, such as food and warmth. He also took a longer view, believing certain fundamentals of our physical appearance could be changed, as in his essay on *How to Grow Tall*:

'Men of different races vary as to average height; the Esquimaux averages 4ft 6in, whilst the Highlander averages about 5ft 10in. Individuals vary as well; we have dwarfs 3ft high and we have giants, if we may so call them, up to 7 or 8 feet. Between these extremes there is a mean, which differs in every country. In the United Kingdom, the Scotch are the tallest; following these are the Irish; the English come next and least of all are the Welsh. The men in the hilly and mountainous districts are taller than those of the same race who live on the plains, and country people are taller than those brought up in towns. Children brought up in open and healthy suburbs are taller than those brought up in the courts and alleys of our large towns. The richer classes are also taller than the poorer – at least in England.

'When we inquire more deeply into this subject, we find that favourable dietetic and hygienic conditions increase growth, whilst wrong foods and unhealthy surroundings cause a dwarfing of both the mind and the body. With regard to food, we notice that flesh foods have a dwarfing influence on mankind, whilst grain foods cause us to attain a good height. The reason of this is due to the fact that flesh is deficient in bone-forming matter and is a poor food generally. Grain foods, on the contrary, are rich in bone-forming material and supply nutriment in a form that is easily digested and absorbed... . This will explain in a great measure the tallness of the Scotchman and the lesser height of the Englishman, because the former feeds largely on oatmeal and the latter eats more meat and other poor and imperfect foods... .

'One of the first conditions for proper growth is the eating of grain foods, such as oats, wheat, barley, maize and other grains and they must be entire – the bran or insoluble matter must not be taken away. Macaroni, vermicelli, semolina and the various preparations of wheat help men to grow tall but to get the best results the entire grain must be eaten. Fruits, vegetables and greenstuffs do not seem to be of much value as height inducers. Milk in moderation is useful. Regular exercise of all the muscles favours growth, but excessive and too early use of the bodily powers tends to stunt growth. Pure air also helps one to gain a proper stature, as it enables the body to burn up waste and carry on life more briskly. Light has a beneficial influence. The more sunlight and daylight a person gets, the more chance has he of growing tall.'

How to become beautiful and attractive

Allinson went further even than height. In an essay that would, had it been published today, surely been a runaway bestseller, he promises his readers *How to Become Beautiful and Attractive*. This gives some surprising insights into the world of Victorian beauty regimes – charcoal for teeth cleaning and eating to attain the correct plumpness may seem unlikely today. But then Allinson would have probably not thought much of Twenty-First Century fashions either. Our models would definitely be classified under 'scragginess' and our shoes would be universally banned on health grounds. He does not, however, regard his beauty tips as a mere sop to vanity, as his introduction explains:

'I consider it the duty of all persons to makes themselves as comely and beautiful as possible. Pretty things in nature are always admired and searched for. In the same way handsome people are usually sought after more than plain and common ones, unless the latter have some other attraction which draws more than a beautiful appearance. When Nature fails, art steps in and tries to imitate it, but such deception is readily detected, as only a patchwork on the original. We find the prettiest women among the peasantry who live simply and breathe pure air. The Irish poor are noted for their beauty, but their lives are not made comfortable by the things that money brings. The special points of attraction are the face, figure, hands and feet. People's idea of beauty varies very much according to their country, education and surroundings; but all are agreed that health is necessary to good looks.

'The Face: This should be free from blotches, pimples, blackheads and eruptions. The skin should be clearly, slightly transparent, have a rose hue and a healthy redness over the cheeks. A face like this is sure to attract wherever it goes. Blotches, pimples and eruptions of all kinds are brought on by wrong living; butter, sugar, jams, preserves, grease, fatty and fried things all tend to bring them out; want of pure air, exercise and bathing also favours their appearance. A dirty grimy appearance of the skin is generally caused by the same wrong foods and habits. A pale yellowish skin with whitish lips most often indicates anaemia or bloodlessness, to cure which proper food, regular exercise, the daily bath and pure air are requisite. Excessive redness, a kind of raw appearance on the cheeks shows eczema; the cure for this condition is the same as for pimples. To keep the skin of the face soft and fine, it should be washed daily or twice a day with tepid or cold water, but soap must not be used. Even the best soaps irritate the skin and are likely to make it rough, it is only when the skin is very grimey that soap should be used. The best thing to remove dirt or use for the face is fine oatmeal. A small jar of this may be kept on the washing stand. After washing the hands with any good soap, a little oatmeal is placed in the palm of the hand, a few drops of water are added and a paste formed; this should be rubbed over the face and neck freely and must be removed with a good sluicing of water. To dry the face, a soft towel is required, as a rough one irritates the delicate skin. Two towels may be kept on the stand – a fine one for the face and a rough one for the skin of the body. Soap applied to the face often makes it shiny, as if it had been polished. The oatmeal cannot well be used by men with beards as it gets amongst the hair and is difficult to remove.

'The teeth as part of the face must not be overlooked. They should be brushed at least once a day with a soft tooth brush. The best thing to clean them with is soap or precipitated chalk; other things are not so good; powdered pumice stone and charcoal are positively injurious. Decayed teeth should be stopped as they are unsightly and taint the breath; those lost should be replaced by artificial ones. The teeth supplied by a good dentist improve the appearance, make the speech clear and assist the proper mastication of food.

'A question I am being often asked is how to remove superfluous hairs which will grow on some ladies' upper lips or other parts of the face. Various pastes are advertised, but they only destroy the hair above the surface, it grows again and the substance used always irritates the skin and may spoil it. Plucking them out or shaving does not cure. Within the last few years a way of permanently removing them by electricity has been discovered. It is almost painless, leaves no scars and the hairs do not grow back again. This is called electrolysis and is now done by lady operators.

'**The Figure**: The lines of Nature cannot be improved by art. All artists consider the natural contours and curves of the human figure to be beautiful in themselves and for us mortals to try to improve upon them is time mis-spent. The fashion of drawing in the waist to make it look waspish is both ungraceful and injurious. I look upon corsets as an evil invention, whereby woman is led to physical destruction. Whoever invented stays deserves to have his name held up to infamy for all ages. They are a curse and cause women more aches, pains, ill health, sickness and premature decay than people are aware of. They train the figure up to an artificial standard, which is not graceful or artistic, but only fashionable, while they produce serious physical evils. If women want to compete with men on an equal footing, they must throw aside these things. As long as women try and ensnare (I mean this word) men by such waists, they must expect to be man's toy and plaything, but not his equal and helpmate. I desire to see woman man's equal, able to hold her own, and not merely his slave to be fed or starved at his caprice. Now, women, will you be free or remain in bondage? Remember: corsets produce ill health by compressing the abdominal organs; the chest cannot be properly expanded, as we find a woman without them can breathe a third more air than one with them on. Hence women who wear them do not get sufficient pure air, their blood is not purified enough and they suffer from cold hands and feet, chilblains, red noses &c, when the cold weather sets in. Corsets often press the nipple into the breasts and so cause trouble when a woman has to suckle her baby.... .

'The figure may be too stout or too thin. Stoutness is very unsightly and takes away all the charm from a woman. To overcome this, limiting food, avoiding sugar, potatoes, rice, jam, preserves, fat, grease and stimulants are necessary; much fluid also tends to keep up this condition. Thinness (or scragginess, so called) may be overcome by careful living, by plain but wholesome foods and obedience to hygienic rules. Rice, sago, tapioca, macaroni and other puddings, potatoes, carrots, turnips and artichokes, help to put on flesh; but greasy foods should be eaten with caution, as these may not add weight without causing pimples as well. The food should be eaten cool and well chewed, then it will nourish the body; much drink should not be taken at meal times, but a little to drink an hour afterwards, if required. Tea and coffee are not good for the thin, as they cause more or less indigestion; cocoa or milk and water are to be preferred.

'Need I remind ladies that a daily sponge bath is most necessary. If they perspire much they must have a morning wash or the armpits become very unpleasant and strong. Plain food, no stimulants, obedience to hygienic rules and a daily sponge will cure this.

'The hands may be kept soft by using gloves when doing rough and dirty work. To cleanse the hands use a good soap and thoroughly dry afterwards with a soft towel. Chapped hands and hands on which large cracks come, show that the person suffers from eczema, of which cracks are a symptom. This must be remedied by plenty of fruit, vegetables and greenstuff; sugar, sweet things and rich foods must be eaten sparingly. Exercise and fresh air must be taken regularly. Chilblains which disfigure the hands during winter come on mainly because enough exercise is not taken; the cure is daily sharp exercise of two or three hours. The nails should be kept clean and not allowed to grow too long; to keep the flesh from growing down them, push it back with the towel after washing the hands. Gloves keep the hands soft, white and clean and those who want to have such hands should wear them regularly.

'The feet should be treated rationally. Boots with wide toes and low heels should be worn and if they fit properly there will be no corns.

The best remedy for corns is a bit of plaister of any kind that softens the corn and then it can be picked out. Blisters on the feet are caused by ill-fitting boots; they should be pricked. In-growing toe nail is caused by compress of the toe by pointed shoes. The remedy is to cut the nail down the side; caustic is a useless torture…. . Persons who suffer from perspiring feet must avoid all sweet foods and drinks and all fatty and rich foods… . Heavy boots and shoes must be worn as little as possible and low shoes or slippers when at home. Now my readers know how to become healthy, beautiful and attractive.'

How to improve memory

It wasn't just the face, the height or the body that Allinson could improve, however, his powers reached even to the brain itself. In his essay *How to Improve the Memory*, he has a few recommendations:

'A good memory is necessary for anyone who wants to succeed in life; on it many things turn and on remembrance of various details success or failure often hangs. I need not dwell on what memory is, but state that he who can remember well caries out his work in a proper manner and leaves nothing undone.

'Memory, as we know, depends on two things – first a system in good condition; secondly a proper mode of observing things; the distinction, in fact, between "eyes and no eyes". That memory is greatly dependent on good health I see every day; a complaint I often hear in my consulting room or read in the numerous letters I receive is loss of memory, inability to fix the attention and no interest in the work the patients are doing. The use of drugs and of things that are not foods are the most common cause of bad memory; poisons like morphia, belladonna, bromide of potassium &c deaden the recalling powers very greatly; alcohol, tobacco, tea and coffee do it in a less degree. Want of exercise leaves the system in a weak condition and the facts learned or observations made, do not get stamped hard enough on the brain and so are soon lost. Impure air makes us feel tired and sleepy and we cannot apply ourselves sufficiently closely to our studies to get a firm grasp of the subject without which a good memory is impossible. Working too many hours without a break tires the brain; the facts then learned rest lightly on the mind and are not easily recalled.

'A bad memory may also be due to inattention to our work. Thus, when a person is learning anything he must throw himself into his work if he means to remember it. Those who wish to get anything by heart must repeat it again and again until the mind can recall it easily. Better still, if a learner can connect the various parts of the subject together, one part follows another and the whole is remembered. Where dry facts have to be mastered there is nothing like writing them down; this is equal in value to reading a thing over half a dozen times. The secret of memory is to make the unfamiliar, familiar; the familiar more familiar; and to connect all things together as much as possible.

'**NB**: Above all things, there must be no deadening of the various mental faculties by alcoholic liquors, tea, coffee and tobacco. This last poison, an Irishman once said "enabled him to think of nothing". This he said when praising it.'

PART FOUR: RECIPES

THOMAS Allinson extended his practical advice even into the kitchen, producing *The Allinson Vegetarian Cookery Book of 1915* to promote his rules of hygienic living. While in most of his essays, he recommends the plainest of food – bread and fruit probably being his favourite meal – here he suggests rather more elaborate fare. The mainstay is, as ever, of course, wholemeal flour as explains in his introduction:

'Throughout this book it will be found that the use of wholemeal has been introduced in the place of white flour. Those persons who do not care to follow the hygienic principle in its entirety can easily substitute white flour if preferred. The recipes have been written bearing in mind the necessity for a wholesome diet; and they will be found to be less rich than those in most of the cookery books published. Should any one wish to make the dishes richer, it can easily be done by an addition of butter, eggs, or cream.

'Let me draw the attention of vegetarians to the use of soaked sago in many dishes. This is a farinaceous food which should be used much more largely in vegetarian cookery than it is. Thoroughly soaked sago should be used in all dishes, savouries or sweets, in which a substitute for suet is required to lighten the mixture; that is, in boiled savouries or sweets which are largely made of wholemeal, as, for instance, in vegetable haggis, roly-poly pudding, and all fruit or vegetable puddings which are boiled in a paste. When soaked sago is used (taking a teacupful of dry sago to two breakfastcupfuls of meal) a light paste will be obtained which would mislead any meat eater into the belief that suet or, at any rate, baking powder had been used. Baking powder, tartaric acid, soda and bicarbonate of soda, are all most injurious to the system, and these chemicals have been left out of this book entirely. In breads and cakes I have used a small quantity of yeast for the rising of the dough; those who once have got accustomed to the use of yeast will not find it any more trouble than using baking powder. It may here be beneficial to give a few hints as to the harm done by the use of the most commonly introduced chemicals, namely, soda, bicarbonate of soda, baking powder, tartaric acid, and citric acid. Not only do they delay the digestion of the foods in which they are used, and give rise to various stomach troubles, but also cause rheumatism and gout, and often are the primary cause of stone in the kidney and bladder. Another danger lies in the fact that these chemicals are too dear to be supplied pure to the public, which always demands cheap goods, and the result is that many of the chemicals in the market are mixed with other still worse poisons, like arsenic, for instance. Self-raising flour, which is liked by so many on account of its convenience, is nothing but ordinary flour mixed with some sort of baking powder; in the same way egg powders are simply starch powders, coloured and flavoured, mixed with baking powder. Tartaric acid and citric acid also belong to the class of injurious chemicals. They are often used in the making of acid drinks, when lemons are not handy. They irritate the stomach violently, and often cause acute dyspepsia. These few remarks will, I hope, convince the readers that all these chemicals are best avoided in culinary preparations. Even salt and spices are best used in great moderation; if our dishes could be prepared without them it would be far the best; but it takes a long time to wean people entirely from the use of condiments; the first step towards it is to use them as sparingly as possible.

'I have tried to make this a hygienic cookery book; but there are a number of dishes introduced which can hardly claim to be hygienic; it has to be left to the good judgment of the readers to use them on rare occasions only, and it will be better for the health of each individual if the plainer dishes only are prepared for the daily table. I wish here to impress on vegetarians, and those who wish to give the diet a trial, not to eat much pulse; this is the rock on which many 'would-be vegetarians' come to grief. They take these very concentrated, nitrogenous foods in rather large quantities, because they have an idea that only they will support them when the use of meat is abandoned. They are foods which, to be beneficial to the system of the consumer, require a great deal of muscular exertion on his part. The results to persons of sedentary habits of eating pulse foods often are indigestion, heavy and dull feelings, and general discomfort. In my own household butter beans, the most concentrated of all foods, come on the table perhaps once a month, lentils or peas perhaps once a week. None but those persons who have strong digestive organs should eat pulse foods at all; and then only when they have plenty of physical work to do. I have known several people who tried vegetarianism who have given up the trial in despair, and, when I inquired closely into the causes, the abuse of pulse food was generally the chief one.

'I now leave this book in the hands of the public. I hope that it will be found useful by many and a help to those who wish to live in a way which is conducive to health and at the same time innocent of slaughter and cruelty. The health of the nation to a great extent is in the hands of our cooks and housewives. If they learn to prepare wholesome and pure food, those who are dependent on them will benefit by it. Healthful cookery must result in health to the household and, therefore, to the nation. Avoid disease-communicating foods, use those only which are conducive to health, and you will be rewarded by an increase of health and consequently of happiness.'

Chapter 1

SOUPS AND STEWS

ARTICHOKE SOUP

1lb each of artichokes [Jerusalem] and potatoes, 1 Spanish onion, 1oz of butter, 1 pint of milk, and pepper and salt to taste.

Peel, wash, and cut into dice the artichokes, potatoes, and onion. Cook them until tender in 1 quart of water with the butter and seasoning. When the vegetables are tender rub them through a sieve. Return the liquid to the saucepan, add the milk, and boil the soup up again. Add water if the soup is too thick. Serve with Allinson plain rusks, or small dice of bread fried crisp in butter or vege-butter.

BARLEY SOUP

8oz of pearl barley, 2 onions, 4 potatoes, 1/2 a teaspoonful of thyme, 1 dessertspoonful of finely chopped parsley, 3 1/2 pints of water, 1/2 pint of milk, 1oz of butter.

Pick and wash the barley, chop up the onions, slice the potatoes. Boil the whole gently for 4 hours with the water, adding the butter, thyme, pepper and salt to taste. When the barley is quite soft, add the milk and parsley, boil the soup up, and serve.

BREAD SOUP

1/2lb of stale crusts of Allinson wholemeal bread, 4 onions, 2 turnips, 1 stick of celery, 1oz of butter, 1/2oz of finely chopped parsley, 8 pints of water, 1/2 pint of milk.

Soak the crusts in the water for 2 hours before they are put over the fire. Cut up into small dice the vegetables; add them to the bread with the butter and pepper and salt to taste. Allow all to simmer gently for 1 hour, then rub the soup through a sieve, return it to the saucepan, add the milk and parsley, and, if the flavour is liked, a little grated nutmeg; boil the soup up and serve at once.

CARROT SOUP

4 good-sized carrots, 1 head of celery, 1 onion, 3oz of Allinson wholemeal bread without crust, 1oz. of butter, pepper and salt, and 1 blade of mace.

Wash, scrape, and cut the carrots into dice. Prepare and cut up the onions and celery. Set the vegetables over the fire with 3 pints of water, adding the mace and seasoning. Let all cook until quite soft, which will probably be in 1–1/2 hours. If the carrots are old, they will take longer cooking. When the vegetables are tender, rub all through a sieve, return the soup to the saucepan, add the butter, allow it to boil up, and serve with sippets of toast.

CLEAR SOUP (with Dumplings)

2 large English onions, 1 teaspoonful of herbs, 1/2 teaspoonful of nutmeg, 1 carrot, 1 turnip, pepper and salt to taste, 1oz of butter, 3 pints of water.

Chop up finely the onions and fry them brown in the butter in the saucepan in which the soup is to be made; add the water. Cut up in thin slices the carrot and turnip, add these, with the herbs, nutmeg, and seasoning to the soup. Let it boil for 1 hour, drain the liquid, return it to the saucepan, and when boiling add the dumplings prepared as follows:

1/2 pint of clear soup, 4 eggs, a little nutmeg, pepper and salt to taste.

Beat the eggs well, mix them with the soup, and season the mixture with nutmeg, pepper, and salt. Pour it into a buttered jug; set it in a pan with boiling water, and let the mixture thicken. Then cut off little lumps with a spoon, and throw these into the soup and boil up before serving.

LENTIL SOUP

1lb each of lentils and potatoes, 1 large Spanish onion, 1 medium-sized head of celery (or the outer pieces of a head of celery, saving the heart for table use), 1 breakfastcupful of tinned tomatoes or 1/2lb. of fresh ones, 1oz. of butter, pepper and salt to taste.

Chop the onion up roughly, and fry it in the butter until beginning to brown. Pick and wash the lentils, and set them over the fire with 2 quarts of water or vegetable stock, adding the fried onion. Peel, wash, and cut up the potatoes, prepare the celery, cut it into small pieces, and add all to the lentils. When they are nearly soft add the tomatoes. When all the ingredients are quite tender rub them through a sieve. Return the soup to the saucepan, add pepper and salt, and more water if the soup is too thick. Serve with sippets of toast.

MACARONI STEW

6 oz of cold boiled macaroni*, 1 large Spanish onion, 1 carrot, 1/2lb of tomatoes, 1/2lb of mushrooms, 2oz of grated cheese, 1oz of butter, pepper and salt to taste.

Wash, prepare, and cut up the vegetables in small pieces. Cover them with water and stew them until tender, adding the butter and seasoning. When tender add the macaroni cut into finger lengths, and the cheese.

* Allinson uses macaroni to mean any kind of pasta

MILK SOUP

2 onions, 2 turnips, I head of celery, 3 pints of milk, I pint of water, 2 tablespoonfuls of Allinson fine wheatmeal, pepper and salt to taste.

Chop up the vegetables and boil them in the water until quite tender. Rub them through a sieve, return the whole to the saucepan, add pepper and salt, rub the wheatmeal smooth in the milk, let the soup simmer for 5 minutes, and serve.

SPANISH SOUP

3 pints of chestnuts peeled and skinned, 2 Spanish onions, 6 potatoes, 2 turnips cut up in dice, I teaspoonful of thyme, I dessertspoonful of vinegar, 2oz of grated cheese, Ioz of butter, 2 quarts of water, pepper and salt to taste.

Boil the chestnuts and vegetables gently until quite tender, which will take I 1/2 hours. Rub them through a sieve and return the soup to the saucepan; add the butter; vinegar and pepper and salt to taste. Let it boil 10 minutes, and sift in the cheese before serving.

Chapter 2

SAVOURIES

CAULIFLOWER AND POTATO PIE

1 fair-sized boiled (cold) cauliflower, 1lb of cold boiled potatoes, 1 pint of milk, 3 eggs, 8oz of Allinson fine wheatmeal, 1 1/2 oz of butter, 4oz of grated cheese, pepper and salt to taste.

Cut up the cauliflower and potatoes, sprinkle half the cheese between the vegetables, make a batter of the milk and eggs and meal, add seasoning to it, place the vegetables in a pie-dish, pour the batter over them, cut the butter into little bits and put them on the top of the pie, sprinkle the rest of the cheese over all, and bake for 1 hour.

COLCANON

1 large cabbage, 1 pint of mashed potatoes, 2oz of grated cheese, 2 eggs, 1oz of butter, 1/2 saltspoonful of nutmeg, pepper and salt to taste.

Boil the cabbage in 1 pint of water until quite tender, drain the water off to keep for stock, chop the cabbage up fine; mix it with the mashed potatoes, the butter and seasoning and the grated cheese; beat up the eggs, and mix these well with the rest; press the mixture into a greased mould, heat all well through in the oven or in a steamer, turn out and serve with a white sauce. This can be made from cold potatoes and cold cabbage.

CORN PUDDING

I tin of sweet corn, I pint of milk, 4 eggs, oz of butter, 8oz of Allinson fine wheatmeal, $^1/_2$ saltspoonful of nutmeg, pepper and salt to taste.

Make a batter of the meal, eggs and milk, add the other ingredients, pour the mixture into a pie-dish, and let it bake I hour.

CURRY SAVOURY

I breakfastcupful of rice, I ditto of Egyptian lentils, Ilb of tomatoes, I dessertspoonful of curry [powder], 2 eggs well beaten, Ioz of butter, salt to taste.

Boil the rice and lentils together until quite tender, and let them cool a little. Slice the tomatoes into a pie-dish, mix the curry, eggs, and salt with the rice and lentils, add a little milk if necessary; spread the mixture over the tomatoes, with the butter in bits over the top, and bake the savoury from $^1/_2$ to I hour.

HAGGIS

2oz of wheatmeal, Ioz of rolled oatmeal, I egg, $^1/_2$oz of oiled butter, $^1/_2$lb small sago, 3 eggs, I large Spanish onion, I dessertspoonful of mixed powdered herbs, Ioz of butter, pepper and salt to taste, and a little milk if needed.

Swell the sago over the fire with as much water as it will absorb; when quite soft put into it the butter to melt, and, when melted, mix in the oatmeal and wheatmeal. Grate the onion, and whip up the eggs; mix all the ingredients together, not forgetting the herbs and seasoning. The whole should be a thick porridgy mass; if too dry add a little milk. Butter a pudding basin, pour into it the mixture, place a piece of buttered paper over it, tie a pudding cloth over the basin, and steam the haggis for 3 hours.

HERB PIE

1 handful of parsley, 1 handful of spinach, and 1 of mustard and cress, 2 lettuce hearts sliced fine, 2 small onions, and a little butter, 3 eggs, 1 pint of milk, and 1/2lb of Allinson fine wheatmeal.

Chop all the vegetables up finely, and mix them with a batter made of the milk, meal, and eggs; season it with pepper and salt; mix well; pour the mixture into a buttered pie-dish, place bits of butter over the top, and bake it for 1 1/2 hours.

HOT-POT

2lbs of potatoes, 3/4lb of onions, 1 breakfastcupful of tinned tomatoes, or 1/2lb of sliced fresh ones, 1 teaspoonful of thyme, 1 1/2oz butter, pepper and salt to taste.

Those who do not like tomatoes can leave them out, and the dish will still be very savoury. The potatoes should be peeled, washed, and cut into thin slices, and the onions peeled and cut into thin slices. Arrange the vegetables and tomatoes in layers; dust a little pepper and salt between the layers, and finish with a layer of potatoes. Cut the butter into little bits, place them on the top of the potatoes, fill the dish with hot water, and bake the hot-pot for 2 hours or more in a hot oven. Add a little more hot water if necessary while baking to make up for what is lost in the cooking.

LEEK PIE

1 bunch of leeks, 1lb of potatoes, 1/2 teaspoonful of herbs, a little nutmeg, 1 pint of milk, pepper and salt to taste, 8oz of Allinson fine wheatmeal, 3 eggs, 1oz of butter.

Cut up into dice the potatoes and leeks, parboil them in 1 pint of water, adding the herbs, butter, and seasoning; place the vegetables in a pie-dish, make a batter with the milk, eggs, and meal, pour it over the vegetables, mix all well, and bake the pie 1 1/2 to 2 hours in a moderate oven.

LENTIL RISSOLES

1/2lb of lentils, 1 finely chopped onion, 1 breakfastcupful of breadcrumbs, 1 breakfastcupful of tinned tomatoes, 1 1/2oz of butter, 2 eggs, pepper and salt to taste, some raspings, butter, vege-butter or oil for frying.

Pick and wash the lentils, and boil them in enough water to cover them; when this is absorbed add the tomatoes, and if necessary gradually a little more water to prevent the lentils from burning. Fry the onion in 1 1/2oz of butter, mix it with the lentils as they are stewing, and add pepper and salt to taste. When the lentils are quite soft, and like a pureé (which will take from 1 to 1 1/2 hours), set them aside to cool. Mix the lentils and the breadcrumbs, beat up one of the eggs and add it to the mixture, beating all well together. If it is too dry, add a very little milk, but only just enough to make the mixture keep together. Form into rissoles, beat up the second egg, roll them into the egg and raspings*, and fry the rissoles a nice brown in boiling butter or oil. Drain and serve.

* raspings are finely ground breadcrumbs

MUSHROOM CUTLETS

1/2lb of mushrooms, 1/2 teacupful of mashed potatoes, 1 teacupful of breadcrumbs, 1 small onion, 2 eggs, 2oz of butter, a little milk, 1 teaspoonful of finely chopped parsley, 1/2 teaspoonful of herbs. Peel and cut up the mushrooms, chop up the onion, and fry them in 1oz of butter.

Mix the mushrooms and onion with the breadcrumbs, 1 egg well beaten, add also pepper and salt to taste; if necessary add a little milk to make it into a paste; shape the mixture into cutlets, dip them in the other egg well beaten, and fry them in the rest of the butter. Serve with tomato sauce.

ONION TURNOVER

2 medium-sized Spanish onions, 1oz of butter (or Allinson frying oil), 3 eggs, pepper and salt. For the pastry, 6oz of Allinson fine wheatmeal, $2^1/2$oz of butter or oil.

Chop the onions fine, boil them a few minutes in a little water, and drain them; stew them in the butter for 10 minutes, adding the seasoning beat up the eggs and mix them well with the onions over the fire, remove the mixture as it begins to set. Have ready the pastry made with the meal, butter, and a little cold water, roll it out, place the onions and eggs on it, fold the pastry over, pinching the edges over, and bake the turnover brown. Serve with gravy. This is a Turkish dish.

POTATO PIE

Slice potatoes and onions, stew with a little water until nearly done, put into a pie-dish, flavour with herbs, pepper, and salt, add a little soaked tapioca and very little butter, cover with short wheatmeal crust, and bake 1 hour. To make a very plain pie-crust use about 2oz of butter or a proportionate quantity of Allinson frying oil to 1lb of wheatmeal. Roll or touch with the fingers as little as possible, and mix with milk instead of water. Eat this pie with green vegetables.

TOMATOES À LA PARMESAN

4 large tomatoes, 1oz of butter, 3oz of Parmesan cheese, $1/2$ pint of milk, 1 dessertspoonful of Allinson fine wheatmeal, pepper and salt to taste.

Bake the tomatoes in a tin with the butter and a dredging of pepper and salt. Make a sauce with the milk, meal, and cheese, seasoning it with a little cayenne pepper if handy. When the tomatoes are baked, place them on hot buttered toast, pour the sauce over, and serve hot.

NUTROAST

1lb breadcrumbs, 6oz ground cob nuts, 2oz butter (oiled), 4 eggs; 1 small onion chopped very fine, 1 good pinch of mixed herbs, pepper and salt to taste, and enough milk just to smoothly moisten the mixture.

Mix all the ingredients thoroughly, turn into a buttered bread tin and steam 2^1/2–3 hours; turn out and serve with brown sauce.

CURRIED RICE AND TOMATOES

^{1}/2lb of Patna rice, 1 dessertspoonful of curry powder, salt to taste, and 1oz of butter.

Wash the rice; mix 1 pint of cold water with the curry powder, put this over the fire with the rice, butter, and salt. Cover the rice with a piece of buttered paper and let it simmer gently until the water is absorbed. This will take about 20 minutes. Rice cooked this way will have all the grains separate. For the tomatoes proceed as follows: 1lb of tomatoes and a little butter, pepper and salt. Wash the tomatoes and place them in a flat tin with a few spoonfuls of water; dust them with pepper and salt, and place little bits of butter on each tomato. Bake them from 15 to 20 minutes, according to the size of the tomatoes and the heat of the oven. Place the rice in the centre of a hot flat dish, put the tomatoes round it, pour the liquid over the rice, and serve.

Chapter 3

VEGETABLES

I HAVE not given recipes for the cooking of plain greens, as they are prepared very much alike everywhere in England. There are a number of recipes in this book giving savoury ways of preparing them, and I will now make a few remarks on the cooking of plain vegetables. The English way of boiling them is not at all a good one, as most of the soluble vegetable salts, which are so important to our system, are lost through it. Green vegetables are generally boiled in a great deal of salt water; this is drained off when they are tender, and the vegetables then served. A much better way for all vegetables is to cook them in a very small quantity of water, and adding a small piece of butter (1oz to 2lb of greens) and a little salt. When the greens are tender, any water which is not absorbed should be thickened with a little Allinson fine wheatmeal and eaten with the vegetables. A great number of them, such as cabbages, savoys, Brussel sprouts, Scotch kail, turnip-tops, &c., can be prepared this way.

In the case of vegetables like asparagus, cauliflower, sea kale, parsnips, artichokes, carrots or celery, which cannot always be stewed in a little water, this should be saved as stock for soups or sauces. Most of these vegetables are very nice with a white sauce; carrots are particularly pleasant with parsley sauce.

Spinach is a vegetable which English cooks rarely prepare nicely; the Continental way of preparing it is as follows: The spinach is cooked without water, with a little salt; when quite tender it is strained, turned on to a board, and chopped very finely; then it is returned to the saucepan with a piece of butter, a little nutmeg, or a few very finely chopped eschalots and some of the juice previously strained. When the spinach is cooking a little Allinson fine wheatmeal, smoothed in 1 or 2 tablespoonfuls of milk, is added to bind the spinach with the juice; cook it a few minutes longer, and serve it with slices of hard-boiled egg on the top.

Potatoes also require a good deal of care. When peeled, potatoes are plainly boiled, they should be placed over the fire after the water has been strained; the potatoes should be lightly shaken to allow the moisture to steam out. This makes them mealy and more palatable. Potatoes which have been baked in their skins should be pricked when tender, or the skins be cracked in some way, otherwise they very soon become sodden. A very palatable way of serving potatoes, is to peel them and bake them in a tin with a little oil or butter, or vege-butter; they should be turned occasionally, in order that they should brown evenly. This is not a very hygienic way of preparing potatoes. From a health point of view they are best baked in their skins, or steamed with or without the skins.

A good many vegetables may be steamed with advantage; for instance, cabbage, sprouts, turnips, parsnips, swedes, Scotch kail, &c. Any way of preparing greens is better than boiling them in a large saucepanful of water and throwing this away. I may just mention that Scotch kail, after being boiled in a little water, should be treated exactly as spinach, and is most delicious in that way; an onion cooked with it greatly improves the flavour.

CARROTS WITH PARSLEY SAUCE

Scrub and wash as many carrots as are required. Cook them in a little water or steam them until quite tender, then slice them and place them in a saucepan. The sauce is made thus: 1 pint of milk, 1 tablespoonful of Allinson wholemeal, a handful of finely chopped parsley, the juice of $1/2$ a lemon, pepper and salt to taste. Boil the milk and thicken it with the meal, which should first be smoothed with a little cold milk, then last of all add the lemon juice, the seasoning, and the parsley. Pour the sauce over the carrots, and let them simmer for ten minutes. Serve very hot with baked potatoes.

CABBAGE

Remove the outer coarse leaves, cut the cabbage in four pieces lengthways, and well wash the pieces in salt water. The salt is added because it kills any insects which may be present. Wash the cabbage as often as is necessary in pure water after this to clean it and remove the salt, and then shred it up fine. Set it over the fire with $1/2$ pint of water, 1oz of butter, a dash of pepper, and a very little salt. Let it cook very gently for 2 hours; when it is quite tender, the liquid can be thickened with a little fine wheatmeal; smooth this with a little milk, or water if milk is not handy; boil it up, and serve.

CAULIFLOWER WITH WHITE SAUCE

Trim the cauliflower, cutting away only the bad and bruised leaves and the coarse part of the stalk. Put it into salt water to force out any insects in the cauliflower. After soaking, wash it well in fresh water and boil quickly until tender, and serve with white sauce.

CELERY (ITALIAN)

2 heads of celery, $1/2$ pint of milk, 1oz of butter, 1 egg, 1 cupful of breadcrumbs, pepper and salt to taste.

Cut up the celery into pieces, boil it in water for 10 minutes; drain it and put it into the stewpan with the milk, $1/2$oz butter, pepper and salt. Simmer the celery gently until tender, put it aside to cool a little, and add the egg well beaten. Butter a shallow dish, strew it well with some of the breadcrumbs, and pour in the celery, sprinkle the rest of the breadcrumbs over the top, put the butter over it in little bits, and bake the celery until brown.

ONION TORTILLA

1lb of Spanish onions, $1 1/2$oz of butter or oil, 3 eggs.

Melt the butter in a frying-pan, slice the onions, and fry them for 10 or 15 minutes, beat the eggs, add them to the onions, season with pepper and salt, and fry the whole a light brown on both sides.

SCOTCH OR CURLY KAIL

Scotch kail is best after there has been frost on it. Wash the kail, and cut away the coarse stalks, boil it for $1^{1}/2$ to 2 hours in a small quantity of water, adding a chopped up onion. Drain it when soft and chop it fine like spinach. Into the saucepan in which the kail was cooked put a piece of butter; melt it, and stir into it 1 tablespoonful of Allinson fine wheatmeal, and brown it very slightly. Then add some of the drained-off kail wafer and stir it smooth with the browned flour. Return the chopped Scotch kail to the saucepan, add pepper and salt to taste; let it cook for a minute, and serve.

CAULIFLOWER AU GRATIN

A fair-sized cauliflower, 1 pint of milk, $1^{1}/2$oz of dried Allinson breadcrumbs, 3oz of cheese, $1^{1}/2$oz of butter, 1 heaped-up tablespoonful of Allinson wholemeal flour, a little nutmeg, and pepper and salt to taste.

Boil the cauliflower until half cooked, cut it into pieces, and place them in a pie-dish. Boil the milk, adding the seasoning, $^{1}/2$oz of the butter, and $^{1}/2$ a saltspoonful of the nutmeg. Thicken with the wholemeal smoothed in a little cold milk or water. Stir in the cheese and pour the sauce over the cauliflower. Shake the breadcrumbs over the top, cut the rest of the butter in bits, and place them over the breadcrumbs. Bake for 20 minutes to $^{1}/2$ an hour, or until the cauliflower is soft.

Chapter 4

EGG COOKERY

EGGS ARE a boon to cooks, especially when dishes are wanted quickly. They enter into a great many savoury and sweet dishes, and few cakes are made without them. They can be prepared in a great variety of ways. Eggs are a good food when taken in moderation. As they are a highly nutritious article of food, they should not be indulged in too freely. Eggs contain both muscle and bone-forming material, in fact everything required for building up the organism of the young bird. The chemical composition of hen's and duck's eggs are as follows:

	Hen's egg	Duck's egg.
Water	74.22	71.11
Nitrogen	12.55	12.24
Fat	12.11	15.49
Mineral matter	1.12	1.16
	100.00	100.00

Eggs take a long time to digest if hard boiled. All the fat of the egg is contained in the yolk, but the white of the egg is pure albumen (or nitrogen) and water. Eggs are most easily digested raw or very lightly boiled, and best cooked thus for invalids. The best way of lightly boiling an egg is to put it in boiling water, set the basin or saucepan on the side of the stove, and let it stand just off the boil for five or six minutes. Eggs often crack when they are put into enough boiling water to well cover them, owing to the sudden expansion of the contents. If they are not covered with water there is less danger of them cracking. One can easily tell stale eggs from fresh ones by holding them up to a strong light. A fresh egg looks clear and transparent, whilst stale ones look cloudy and opaque. There are various ways of preserving eggs for the winter; one of the best is by using the Allinson egg preservative. Another very good way is to have stands made with holes which will hold the eggs. Keep these stands in an airy place in a good current of fresh air, and every week turn the eggs, so that one week they stand the pointed end down, next week the rounded end down.

APPLE SOUFFLÉ

4 eggs, 4 apples, 2oz of castor sugar (or more if the apples are very sour), 1 gill of new milk or half milk and half cream, 1oz of Allinson cornflour, and the juice of 1 lemon.

Pare, cut up, and stew the apples with the sugar and lemon juice until they are reduced to a pulp. Beat them quite smooth, and return them to the stewpan. Smooth the cornflour with the milk, and mix it with the apples, and stir until it boils; then turn the mixture into a basin to cool. Separate the yolks from the whites of the eggs; beat the yolks well, and mix them with the apple mixture. Whisk the whites to a stiff froth, mix them lightly with the rest, and pour the whole into a buttered soufflé tin. Bake for 20 minutes in a moderately hot oven, and serve at once.

CHOCOLATE SOUFFLÉ

5 eggs, 2oz of butter, 3oz of castor sugar, 2 large bars of chocolate, 6oz of the crumb of the bread, and vanilla essence to taste.

Cream the butter, and stir into it gradually the yolks of the eggs, the sugar, and chocolate. Previously soak the bread in milk or water. Squeeze it dry, and add to it the other ingredients. Add vanilla and the whites of the eggs whipped to a stiff froth, and pour the mixture into a buttered pie-dish or cake tin. Bake $^1/2$ of an hour, and serve immediately. If the soufflé is baked in a cake tin, a serviette should be pinned round it before serving.

CURRIED EGGS

6 hard-boiled eggs, 1 medium-sized English onion, 1 cooking apple, 1 teaspoonful of curry powder, 1 dessertspoonful of Allinson fine wheatmeal, 1oz of butter, and salt to taste.

Prepare the onion and apple, chop them very fine, and fry them in the butter in a stewpan until brown. Add $^1/2$ pint of water and a little salt. Smooth the curry and wheatmeal with a little cold water, and thicken the sauce with it. Let it simmer for 10 minutes, then rub through a sieve. Return the sauce to the stewpan, shell the eggs, and heat them up in the sauce; serve very hot on a flat dish.

EGGS À LA BONNE FEMME

4 eggs, 1 Spanish onion, 1oz of butter, 1 teaspoonful of vinegar, and 2 tablespoonfuls of breadcrumbs; pepper and salt to taste.

Peel and slice the onion, and fry it brown in the butter; add the vinegar and seasoning when done. Spread the onion on a buttered dish, break the eggs over them, dust these with pepper and salt, and sprinkle with breadcrumbs. Place a few bits of butter on the top, and bake until the eggs are set, which will only take a few minutes.

STUFFED EGGS

4 hard-boiled eggs, 8 Spanish olives, $^1/2$oz of butter, pepper and salt to taste.

Halve the eggs lengthway, and carefully remove the yolks. Pound these well, and mix them with the olives, which should be previously stoned and minced fine; add the butter and pepper and salt, and mix all well. Fill the whites of the eggs with the mixture. Pour some thick white sauce, flavoured with grated cheese, on a hot dish, and place the eggs on it. Serve hot.

SWEET CREAMED EGGS

To each egg allow 2 tablespoonfuls of cream, or new milk, 1 teaspoonful of strawberry or raspberry and currant jam, 1 thin slice of buttered toast, sugar and vanilla to taste.

Butter as many cups as eggs, reckoning 1 egg for each person. Place the jam in the centre of the cup; beat up the eggs with the cream or milk, sugar and vanilla, and divide the mixture into the cups. Cover each cup with buttered paper, stand the cups in a stew-pan with boiling water, which should reach only half-way up the cups, and steam the eggs until they are set--time from 8 to 10 minutes. Turn the eggs out on the buttered toast, and serve hot or cold.

Chapter 5

SALADS

THESE wholesome dishes are not used sufficiently by English people, for very few know the value of them. All may use these foods with benefit, and two dinners each week of them with Allinson wholemeal bread will prevent many a serious illness. They are natural food in a plain state, and supply the system with vegetable salts and acids in the best form. In winter, salads may be made with endive, mustard and cress, watercress, round lettuces, celery, or celery root, or even finely cut raw red or white cabbage; pepper, salt, oil, and vinegar are added as above. As a second course, milk or bread pudding. Salads are invaluable in cases of gout, rheumatism, gallstones, stone in the kidney or bladder, and in a gravelly condition of the water and impure condition of the system.

CHEESE SALAD

Put some finely shredded lettuce in a glass dish, and over this put some young sliced onions, some mustard and cress, a layer of sliced tomatoes, and two hard-boiled eggs, also sliced. Add salt and pepper, and then over all put a nice layer of grated cheese. Serve with a dressing composed of equal parts of cream, salad oil, and vinegar, into which had been smoothly mixed a little mustard.

CUCUMBER SALAD

Peel and slice a cucumber, mix together $^1/2$ a teaspoonful of salt, $^1/2$ of a teaspoonful of white pepper, and 2 tablespoonfuls of olive oil, stir it well together, then add very gradually 1 tablespoonful of vinegar, stirring it all the time. Put the sliced cucumber into a salad dish, and garnish it with nasturtium leaves and flowers.

ONION SALAD

1 large boiled Spanish onion, 3 large boiled potatoes, 1 teaspoonful of parsley, pepper and salt to taste, juice of 1 lemon, 2 or 3 tablespoonfuls of olive oil.

Slice the onion and potatoes when quite cold, mix well together with the parsley and pepper and salt; add the lemon juice and oil, and mix well once more.

POTATO SALAD

1lb of cold boiled potatoes, 1 small beetroot, some spring onions, olives, 4 tablespoonfuls of vinegar, 2 of salad oil, a little tarragon vinegar, salt, pepper, minced parsley.

Cut the potatoes in small pieces, put these into a salad bowl, cut up the onions and olives, and add them to the potatoes. Mix the vinegar, oil, tarragon vinegar, salt, and pepper well together, pour it into the salad bowl, and stir it well. Garnish with beetroot and parsley.

SPANISH SALAD

Put into the centre of the bowl some cold dressed French beans or scarlet runners, and before serving pour over some good mayonnaise. Garnish the beans with three tomatoes cut in slices and arranged in a circle one overlapping the other.

Chapter 6

POTATO COOKERY

POTATO BIRD'S NEST

A plateful of mashed potatoes, 2lbs of spinach well cooked and chopped, 3 hard-boiled eggs, 1oz of butter.

Fry the mashed potatoes a nice brown in the butter, then place it on a dish in the shape of a ring. Inside this spread the spinach, and place the eggs, shelled, on the top of this. Serve as hot as possible.

POTATO CAKES

3 fair-sized potatoes, 1 egg, 2 tablespoonfuls of Allinson fine wheatmeal, pepper and salt to taste, and a pinch of nutmeg.

Peel, wash, and grate the raw potatoes; beat up the egg and mix it with the potatoes, flour, and seasoning. Beat all well together, and fry the mixture like pancakes in oil or butter.

POTATO CHEESE

6oz of mashed potatoes, 2 lemons, 6oz of sugar, 2oz of butter.

Grate the rind of the lemons and pound it well with the sugar in a mortar, add the potatoes very finely mashed; oil the butter and mix this and the lemon juice with the rest of the ingredients; when all is very thoroughly mixed, fill the mixture in a jar and keep closely covered.

POTATO ROLLS (Spanish)

3 teacupfuls of mashed potatoes, 3 tablespoonfuls of Allinson fine wheatmeal, 18 olives, 1 egg well beaten; seasoning to taste.

Stone the olives and chop them up fine, mix the meal, mashed potato, olive, and egg well together; season with pepper and salt; add a little milk if necessary, make the mixture into rolls 3 inches long, brush them over with a pastry brush dipped in Allinson nut-oil or hot butter and bake them on a floured tin until brown, which will take from 10 to 20 minutes. Serve with brown sauce and vegetables.

POTATO SNOW (a Pretty Dish)

1 1/2lbs of potatoes, 3 hard-boiled eggs, 1 small beetroot.

Boil the potatoes till tender, pass them through a potato masher into a hot dish, letting the mashed potato fall lightly, and piling it up high. Slice the eggs and beetroot, and arrange alternate slices of egg and beetroot round the base of the potato snow. Brown the top with a salamander, or, if such is not handy, with a coal-shovel made red hot.

POTATOES (STUFFED)

6 large potatoes, 1 1/2 breakfastcupfuls of breadcrumbs, 1/2lb of grated English onions, 1 teaspoonful of powdered sage, 1 ditto of finely chopped parsley, 1 egg well beaten, piece of butter the size of a walnut, pepper and salt to taste.

Halve the potatoes, scoop them out, leaving nearly 1 inch of the inside all round. Make a stuffing of the other ingredients, adding a very little milk if the stuffing should be too dry; fill the potatoes with it, tie the halves together, and bake them until done. Serve with brown sauce.

Chapter 7

SAUCES

FLESH-EATERS have the gravy of meat to eat with their vegetables, and when they give up the use of flesh they are often at a loss for a good substitute. Sauces may be useful in more ways than one. When not too highly spiced or seasoned they help to prevent thirst, as they supply the system with fluid, and when made with the liquor in which vegetables have been boiled they retain many valuable salts which would otherwise have been lost. When foods are eaten in a natural condition no sauces are required, but when food is changed by cooking many persons require it to be made more appetising, as it is called. The use of sauces is thus seen to be an aid to help down plain and wholesome food, and being fluid they cause the food to be more thoroughly broken up and made into a porridgy mass before it is swallowed. From a health point of view artificial sauces are not good, but if made as I direct very little harm will result.

Brown Gravy, Fried Onion Sauce, or Herb Gravy must be used with great caution, or not at all by those who are troubled with heartburn, acidity, biliousness, or skin eruptions of any kind.

The water in which vegetables (except cabbage or potatoes) have been boiled is better for making sauces than ordinary water.

APPLE SAUCE

1lb of apples, 1 gill of water, 1¹/₂oz of sugar (or more, according to taste), ¹/₂ a teaspoonful of mixed spice.

Pare and core the apples, cut them up, and cook them with the water until quite mashed up, add sugar and spice. Rub the apples through a sieve, re-heat, and serve. Can also be served cold.

APRICOT SAUCE

$^1/2$lb of apricot jam, $^1/2$ a teaspoonful of Allinson cornflour.

Dilute the jam with $^1/2$ pint of water, boil it up and pass it through a sieve; boil the sauce up, and thicken it with the cornflour. Serve hot or cold.

BROWN GRAVY

Put a tablespoonful of butter or olive oil into a frying-pan or saucepan, make it hot, dredge in a tablespoonful of Allinson fine wheatmeal, brown this, then add boiling water, with pepper and salt to taste. A little mushroom or walnut ketchup may be added if desired. Eat with vegetables or savouries.

CHOCOLATE SAUCE

I bar of Allinson chocolate, $^1/2$ pint of milk, $^1/2$ teaspoonful of cornflour, $^1/2$ teaspoonful of vanilla essence.

Melt the chocolate over the fire with I tablespoonful of water, add the milk, and stir well; when it boils add the cornflour and vanilla. Boil the sauce up, and serve.

CURRANT SAUCE (RED & WHITE)

$^1/2$ pint of both white and red currants, 2ozs of sugar, I gill of water, $^1/2$ a teaspoonful of cornflour.

Cook the ingredients for 10 minutes, rub the fruit through a sieve, re-heat it, and thicken the sauce with the cornflour. Serve hot or cold.

CURRY SAUCE

3 English onions, 1 carrot, 1 good cooking apple, 1 teaspoonful of curry powder, 1/2oz of butter, 1 dessertspoonful of Allinson fine wheatmeal, salt to taste.

Chop up the onions, carrot, and apple, and stew them in 1/2 pint of water until quite tender, adding the curry and salt. When quite soft rub the vegetables well through a sieve; brown the meal in the saucepan in the butter, add the sauce to this, and let it simmer for a few minutes; add a little more water if necessary.

MAYONNAISE SAUCE

1/2 pint of oil, the yolk of 1 egg, the juice of a lemon, 1/2 teaspoonful each of mustard, pepper, and salt.

Place the yolks in a basin, which should be quite cold; work them smooth with a wooden spoon, add the salt, pepper, and mustard, and mix all well. Stir in the oil very gradually, drop by drop; when the sauce begins to thicken stir in a little of the lemon juice, continue with the oil, and so on alternately until the sauce is finished. Be sure to make it in a cool place, also to stir one way only. If you follow directions the sauce may curdle; should this ever happen, do not waste the curdled sauce, but start afresh with a fresh yolk of egg, stirring in a little fresh oil first, and then adding the curdled mixture.

Chapter 8

PUDDINGS

ALMOND PUDDING

4 eggs, 3oz of castor sugar, 4oz of ground sweet almonds, $^1/2$oz of ground bitter almonds.

Whip the whites of the eggs to a stiff froth, mix them lightly with the well-beaten yolks, add the other ingredients gradually. Have ready a well-buttered pie-dish, pour the mixture in (not filling the dish more than three-quarters full), and bake in a moderately hot oven until a knitting needle pushed through comes out clean. Turn the pudding out and serve cold.

APPLE CHARLOTTE

2lbs of cooking apples, 1 teacupful of mixed currants and sultanas, 1 heaped up teaspoonful of ground cinnamon, 2oz of blanched and chopped almonds, sugar to taste, Allinson wholemeal bread, and butter.

Pare, core, and cut up the apples and set them to cook with 1 teacupful of water. Some apples require much more water than others. When they are soft, add the fruit picked and washed, the cinnamon, and the almonds and sugar. Cut very thin slices of bread and butter, line a buttered pie-dish with them. Place a layer of apples over the buttered bread, and repeat the layers of bread and apples until the dish is full, finishing with a layer of bread and butter. Bake from $^1/2$ hour to 1 hour.

APRICOT PUDDING

1 tin of apricots, 6 sponge cakes, $^1/_2$ pint of milk, 2 eggs.

Put the apricots into a saucepan, and let them simmer with a little sugar for $^1/_2$ an hour; take them off the fire and beat them with a fork. Mix with them the sponge cakes crumbled. Beat the eggs up with milk and pour it on the apricots. Pour the mixture into a wetted mould and bake in a hot oven with a cover over the mould for $^1/_2$ an hour. Turn out; serve either hot or cold.

BAKED CUSTARD PUDDING

1 pint of milk, 3 eggs, sugar, vanilla flavouring, nutmeg.

Warm the milk, beat up the eggs with the sugar, pour the milk over, and flavour. Have a pie-dish lined at the edge with baked paste, strain the custard into the dish, grate a little nutmeg over the top, and bake in a slow oven for $^1/_2$ an hour. Serve in the pie-dish with stewed rhubarb.

BREAD PUDDING (STEAMED)

$^1/_2$lb of breadcrumbs, 1 wineglassful of rosewater, 1 pint of milk, 3oz of ground almonds, sugar to taste, 4 eggs well beaten, 1oz of butter (oiled).

Mix all the ingredients, and let them soak for $^1/_2$ an hour. Turn into a buttered mould and steam the pudding for $1^1/_2$ to 2 hours.

CABINET PUDDING

Butter a pint pudding mould and decorate it with preserved cherries, then fill the basin with layers of sliced sponge cakes and macaroons, scattering a few cherries between the layers. Make a pint of custard with Allinson custard powder, add to it 2 tablespoonfuls of raisin wine and pour over the cakes, &c., steam the pudding carefully for three-quarters of an hour, taking care not to let the water boil into it; serve with wine sauce.

CANADIAN PUDDING

To use up cold stiff porridge. Mix the porridge with enough hot milk to make it into a fairly thick batter. Beat up 1 or 2 eggs, 1 egg to a breakfastcupful of the batter, add some jam, stirring it well into the batter, bake 1 hour in a buttered pie-dish.

CHOCOLATE TRIFLE

8 sponge cakes, 3 large bars of chocolate, 1/2 pint of cream, white of 1 egg, 3 inches of stick vanilla, 3oz of almonds blanched and chopped, 2oz of ratafia, 1/2 pint of milk.

Break the sponge cakes into pieces, boil the milk and pour it over them; mash them well up with a spoon. Dissolve half the chocolate in a saucepan with 2 tablespoonfuls of water, and flavour it with 1 inch of the vanilla, split; when the chocolate is quite dissolved remove the vanilla. Have ready a wetted mould, put into it a layer of sponge cake, next spread some of the dissolved chocolate, sprinkle with almonds and ratafias, repeat until you finish with a layer of sponge cake. Grate the rest of the chocolate, whip the cream with the whites of eggs, vanilla, and 1 teaspoonful of sifted sugar; sift the chocolate into the whipped cream. Turn the sponge cake mould into a glass dish, spread the chocolate cream over it evenly, and decorate it with almonds.

CHRISTMAS PUDDING

1lb raisins (stoned), 1lb chopped apples, 1lb currants, 1lb breadcrumbs,

$^1/2$lb mixed peel, chopped fine, 1lb shelled and ground Brazil nuts, $^1/2$lb chopped sweet almonds, 1oz bitter almonds (ground), 1lb sugar, $^1/2$lb butter, $^1/2$oz mixed spice, 6 eggs.

Wash, pick, and dry the fruit, rub the butter into the breadcrumbs, beat up the eggs, and mix all the ingredients together; if the mixture is too dry, add a little milk. Fill some greased basins with the mixture, and boil the puddings from 8 to 12 hours.

COCOANUT PUDDING

10oz of fresh grated cocoanut, 8oz of Allinson breadcrumbs, 4oz of stoned muscatels, chopped small, 3oz of sugar, 3 eggs, 1 pint of milk.

Mix the breadcrumbs, cocoanut; muscatels, sugar, and the butter (oiled); add the yolks of the eggs, well beaten, whip the whites of the eggs to a stiff froth, add these to the mixture just before turning the pudding into a buttered pie-dish; bake until golden brown.

GOLDEN SYRUP PUDDING

This pudding is very much liked and easily made. 10oz of Allinson fine wheatmeal, 3 eggs, 1 pint of milk, $^1/2$lb of golden syrup.

Make a batter with the meal, eggs, and milk; grease a pudding basin, pour into it first the golden syrup, then the batter without mixing them; put over the batter a piece of buttered paper, tie up with a cloth, and steam the pudding in boiling water for $2^1/2$ hours, taking care that no water boils into it. If liked, the juice of $^1/2$ lemon may be added to the syrup and grated rind put in the batter. Before turning the pudding out, dip the pudding basin in cold water for 1 minute.

GREENGAGE SOUFFLÉ

20 greengages, 4 eggs, 3 tablespoonfuls of ground rice, $^1/_2$oz of butter, $^1/_2$ pint of milk, $^1/_2$ a teacupful of water, sugar to taste.

Skin and stone the fruit; blanch and drop (or grind) the kernels; gently cook the greengages in the water with the kernels and sugar. When the fruit has been reduced to a pulp mix in gradually the ground rice, which should have been smoothed previously with the milk; add the butter and let the whole mixture boil up; draw the saucepan from the fire and stir in the yolks of the eggs and then the whites beaten to a stiff froth. Pour the mixture into a well-greased dish, and bake the soufflé, for $^1/_2$ an hour in a brisk oven. Serve immediately.

LEMON PUDDING

1lb breadcrumbs, 3 eggs, 3 lemons, 2oz of sago, 1 pint of milk, 2oz of butter, 8oz of sugar.

Soak the sago well in the milk over the fire, add the butter, letting it dissolve, and mix with it the breadcrumbs, the sugar, the juice of the 3 lemons, and the grated rind of 2. Beat the eggs well, mix all the ingredients thoroughly, and pour the mixture into 2 well-greased pudding basins; steam the puddings for 2 hours, and serve them with stewed fruit or white sauce.

OATMEAL PANCAKES

$^1/_2$lb of fine oatmeal, 4 eggs, 1 pint of milk.

Make a batter of the ingredients, and fry the pancakes in butter, oil, or vege-butter in the usual way. These are very good. Serve with lemon and castor sugar.

VANILLA CHESTNUTS (for Dessert)

1lb of chestnuts, ½lb of sugar, 1 teacupful of water, vanilla to taste.

Boil the chestnuts in plenty of water until tender, but not too soft, that they may not break in peeling. Peel them; simmer the sugar and the teacupful of water for 10 minutes, then add the chestnuts. Allow all to cook gently until the syrup browns, add vanilla and remove the chestnuts from the fire; when sufficiently cool, turn the whole into a glass dish.

WHOLEMEAL BANANA PUDDING

2 teacupfuls of Allinson fine wheatmeal, 3oz of sago, 6 bananas, 1 tablespoonful of sugar, 3 eggs, ½ pint of milk.

Peel the bananas and mash them with a fork. Soak the sago with ½ pint of water, either in the oven or in a saucepan. Make a batter with the eggs, meal, and milk; add the bananas, sugar, and sago, and mix all smoothly. Turn the mixture into a greased mould and steam the pudding for 2 hours.

WINIFRED PUDDING

3oz of butter, 3oz of sugar, 2 eggs, 1oz of Allinson breadcrumbs, the juice of 1 lemon, flavouring, puff paste.

Beat the butter and sugar to a cream, beat in the eggs one at a time. Pour sufficient boiling milk over the breadcrumbs to soak, and add them to the mixture, add the strained lemon juice and flavouring, and mix well together. Border a pie-dish and line with paste; put in the mixture, and bake for about 30 minutes in a moderate oven. Sift a little white sugar over, and serve hot or cold.

CHOCOLATE TARTS

6oz of Allinson fine wheatmeal, 2oz of butter, 2oz of Allinson chocolate (grated), 1 dessertspoonful of sugar, 1/2oz of ground rice, 4 eggs, well beaten, and 1 pint of milk.

Mix the milk with the ground rice, add to it the chocolate smoothly and gradually; stir the mixture over the fire until it thickens, let cool a little and stir in the eggs; make the meal and butter into a paste with a little cold water; line a greased plate with it, and pour the cooled custard into it; bake the tart for 1/2 hour in a moderate oven.

MARLBOROUGH PIE

6 good-sized apples, 1oz of butter, 3 eggs, the juice and rind of 1 lemon, 1 teacupful of milk, sugar to taste, and some paste for crust.

Steam or bake the apples till tender and press them through a sieve while hot, add the butter, and let the mixture cool; beat the yolks of the eggs, add to them the milk, sugar, lemon juice and rind, and add all these to the apples and butter; line a dish with paste, fill it with the above mixture, and bake the pie for 1/2 hour in a quick oven; whip the whites of the eggs stiff, adding a little castor sugar, heap the froth over the pie, and let it set in the oven.

LEMON CREAM (for Cheesecakes)

1lb powdered sugar, 6 yolks of eggs, 4 whites of eggs, juice of 8 lemons, grated rind of 2 lemons, 1/2lb fresh butter.

Put the ingredients into a double boiler and stir over a slow fire until the cream is the consistency of honey.

BLACKBERRY CREAM

1 quart of blackberries, sugar to taste, $^1/_2$ pint of cream, white of 2 eggs.
Mash the fruit gently, put it into a hair-sieve and allow it to drain. Sprinkle the fruit with sugar to make the juice drain more freely; whip the cream and mix with the juice.

ORANGE CREAM

6 oranges, 1 lemon, 7 eggs, 4 to 6oz of sugar (according to taste), 1 dessertspoonful of cornflour, some water.

Take the juice of the oranges and the juice and grated rind of the lemon. Add enough water to the fruit juice to make 1 $^1/_2$ pints of liquid; let this get hot, adding the sugar to it; mix the cornflour smooth with a spoonful of cold water, and thicken the fruit juice with it, letting it boil up for a minute, set aside and let it cool a little; beat the eggs well, and when the liquid has cooled mix them carefully in with it; return the whole over a gentle fire, keep stirring continually until the cream thickens, but take care not to let it boil, as this would curdle it. When cold, serve in custard glasses, or in a glass dish poured over macaroons.

GOOSEBERRY FOOL

Top and tail 1 pint of gooseberries, put into a lined saucepan with sugar to taste and half a small teacupful of water, stew gently until perfectly tender, rub through a sieve, and when quite cold add 1 pint of custard made with Allinson custard powder, which should have been allowed to become cold before being mixed with the fruit. Serve in a glass dish with sponge fingers.

N.B.– Apple fool is made in exactly the same way as above, substituting sharp apples for the gooseberries.

APPLE CAKE

6oz each of Allinson fine wheatmeal and white flour, 4^{1}/2oz of butter, I egg, a little cold water, I^{1}/2lbs of apples, I heaped-up teaspoonful of cinnamon, and 3oz of castor sugar.

Rub the butter into the meal and flour, beat up the egg and add it, and as much cold water as is required to make a smooth paste; roll out the greater part of it ^{1}/2 inch thick, and line a flat buttered tin with it. Pare, core, and cut the apples into thin divisions, arrange them in close rows on the paste point down, leaving I inch of edge uncovered; sift the sugar and cinnamon over the apples; roll out thinly the rest of the paste, cover the apples with it, turn up the edges of the bottom crust over the edges of the top crust, make 2 incisions in the crust, and bake the cake until brown in a moderately hot oven; when cold sift castor sugar over it, slip the cake off the tin, cut into pieces, and serve.

APPLE TART (OPEN)

2lbs of apples, I cupful of currants and sultanas, 2oz of chopped almonds, sugar to taste, I teaspoonful of ground cinnamon or the rind of ^{1}/2 lemon (which latter should be removed after cooking with the apples), 12oz or Allinson fine wheatmeal, and 4^{1}/2oz of butter.

Pare, core, and cut up the apples; stew them in very little water, only just enough to keep from burning; when nearly done add the currants, sultanas, almonds, cinnamon, and sugar; let all simmer together until the apples have become a pulp; let the fruit cool; make a paste of the meal, butter, and a little water; roll it out and line a round, flat dish with it, and brush the paste over with white of eggs; turn the apple mixture on the paste; cut the rest of the paste into strips ^{3}/8 of an inch wide, and lay them over the apples in diamond shape, each I inch from the other, so as to make a kind of trellis arrangement of the pastry. If enough paste is left, lay a thin strip right round the dish to finish off the edge, mark it nicely with a fork or spoon, and bake the tart for ^{3}/4 hour. Serve with white sauce or custard.

A DISH OF SNOW

1 pint of thick apple sauce, sweetened and flavoured to taste (orange or rosewater is preferable), the whites of 3 eggs, beaten to a stiff froth. Mix both together, and serve.

COMPÔTE OF ORANGES AND APPLES

6 oranges, 8 fine sweet apples, 1oz of ground sweet almonds, syrup.

Peel the oranges and the apples, cut them across in thin slices, coring the apples and removing the pips from the oranges. Arrange the fruit into alternate circles in a glass dish, sprinkling the ground almonds between the layers. Boil the rind of 3 oranges, $1/2$ pint of water, 4oz of sugar until the syrup is clear, then strain it and when cold pour over the fruit.

STEWED PEARS AND VANILLA CREAM

Get 1 tin of pears, open it, and turn the contents into an enameled stewpan, add some sugar and liquid cochineal to colour the fruit, and let them stew a few minutes. Take out the pears carefully without breaking them, and let the syrup cook until it is thick. When the pears are cold lay them on a dish with the cores upwards, and with a spoon scoop out the core, and fill the space left with whipped cream flavoured with vanilla and sweetened; sprinkle them with finely shredded blanched almonds or pistachios, and pour the syrup round them.

SWISS CREAMS

4oz of macaroons, a little raisin wine and 1 pint of custard, made with Allinson custard powder; lay the macaroons in a glass dish and pour over enough raisin wine to soak them, make the custard in the usual way, let it cool and then pour over the cakes; when quite cold garnish with pieces of bright coloured jelly.

Chapter 9

BREAD AND CAKES

THE ADVANTAGES OF WHOLEMEAL BREAD

PEOPLE are now concerning themselves about the foods they eat, and inquiring into their properties, composition, and suitability. One food that is now receiving a good deal of attention is bread, and we ought to be sure that this is of the best kind, for as a nation we eat daily a pound of it per head. We consume more of this article of food than of any other, and this is as it ought to be, for bread is the staff of life, and many of the other things we eat are garnishings. It is said we cannot live on bread alone, but this is untrue if the loaf is a proper one; at one time our prisoners were fed on it alone, and the peasantry of many countries live on very little else.

Not many years ago books treating of food and nutrition always gave milk as the standard food, and so it is for calves and babies. Nowadays we use a grain food as the standard, and of all grains wheat is the one which is nearest perfection, or which supplies to the body those elements that it requires, and in best proportions. A perfect food must contain carbonaceous, nitrogenous, and mineral matter in definite quantities; there must be from four to six parts of carbonaceous or heat and force-forming matter to one of nitrogen, and from two to four per cent of mineral matter; also a certain bulk of innutritious matter for exciting secretion, for separating the particles of food so that the various gastric and intestinal juices may penetrate and dissolve out all the nutriment, and for carrying off the excess of the biliary and other intestinal secretions with the fæces.

A grain of wheat consists of an outer hard covering or skin, a layer of nitrogenous matter directly under this, and an inner kernel of almost pure starch. The average composition of wheat is this:

Nitrogen	12
Carbon	72
Mineral Matter	4
Water	12
	100

From this analysis we observe that the nitrogenous matter is to the carbonaceous in the proportion of one-sixth, which is the composition of a perfect food. Besides taking part in this composition, the bran, being in a great measure insoluble, passes in bulk through the bowels, assisting daily laxation – a most important consideration. If wheat is such a perfect food, it must follow that wholemeal bread must be best for our daily use. That such is the case, evidence on every side shows; those who eat it are healthier, stronger, and more cheerful than those who do not, all other things being equal. Wholemeal bread comes nearer the standard of a perfect food than does the wheaten grain, as in fermentation some of the starch is destroyed, and thus the proportion of nitrogen is slightly increased.

The next question is, how shall we prepare the grain so as to make the best bread from it? This is done by grinding the grain as finely as possible with stones, and then using the resulting flour for bread-making. The grain should be first cleaned and brushed, and passed over a magnet to cleanse it from any bits of steel or iron it may have acquired from the various processes it goes through, and then finely ground. To ensure fine grinding, it is always advisable to kiln-dry it first. When ground, nothing must be taken from it, nor must anything be added to the flour, and from this bread should be made. Baking powder, soda, and tartaric acid, or soda and hydrochloric acid, or ammonia and hydrochloric acid, or other chemical agents, must never be used for raising bread, as these substances are injurious, and affect the human system for harm. The only ferment that should be used is yeast; of this the French variety is best. If brewer's yeast is used it must be first well washed, otherwise it gives a bitter flavour to the loaf. A small quantity of salt may be used, but not much, otherwise it adds an injurious agent to the bread.

BUTTER BISCUITS

$1/2$lb butter, 2lbs fine wholemeal flour, $1/2$ pint milk.

Dissolve the butter in the milk, which should be warmed, then stir in the meal and make into a stiff, smooth paste, roll it out very thin, stamp it into biscuits, prick them out with a fork, and bake on tins in a quick oven for 10 minutes.

CINNAMON MADEIRA CAKE

$1/2$lb of fine wheatmeal, $1/2$lb of butter, $1/2$lb of sugar, $1/2$lb of currants and sultanas mixed (washed and picked) 5 eggs, 1 dessertspoonful of ground cinnamon.

Beat the butter to a cream, add the sugar, then the eggs well beaten, the meal fruit and cinnamon. Line a cake tin with buttered paper, and bake the cake in a moderate oven from 1 to $1 1/2$ hours.

COCOANUT BISCUITS

2 breakfastcupfuls of wheatmeal, 2 teacupfuls of grated cocoanut, 3 dessertspoonfuls of sugar, 3 tablespoonfuls of orange water, 2oz of butter, a little milk.

Mix the ingredients, adding a little milk to moisten the paste, mix it well, roll the paste out $1/2$ in thick, cut out with a biscuit cutter. Prick the biscuits, and bake them in a moderate oven until a pale brown.

CRISP OATMEAL CAKES

1lb of oatmeal, 2oz of butter or oil (1 tablespoonful of oil is 1oz), 1 gill of cold milk.

Make a dough of the butter, meal, and milk; shake meal plentifully on the board, turn the dough on to it, and having sprinkled this too with meal, work it a little with the backs of your fingers. Roll the dough out to the thickness of a crown piece, cut it in shapes, put the cakes on a hot stove, and when they are a little brown on the underside, take them off and place them on a hanger in front of the fire in order to brown the upper side; when this is done they are ready for use.

DYSPEPTICS' BREAD

9oz of Allinson wholemeal, 1 egg, a scant $1/2$ pint of milk and water.

Separate the yolk from the white of the egg. Beat up the yolk with the milk and water, and mix this with the meal into a thick batter; whip up the white of the egg stiff, and mix it well into the batter. Grease and heat a bread tin, turn the mixture into it, and bake the loaf for $1 1/2$ hours in a hot oven. This is very delicious bread, very light and digestible.

DOUGHNUTS

$1 1/2$lbs of wheatmeal, $1/2$oz yeast, 1 egg, 1 teaspoonful of cinnamon, 3 tablespoonfuls of sugar, enough lukewarm milk to moisten the dough, some jam and marmalade.

Dissolve the yeast in a little warm milk, mix all the ingredients, adding the dissolved yeast and enough milk to make the dough sufficiently moist to handle. Let it rise $1 1/2$ hours in front of the stove. When risen roll it out $1/2$ in thick, cut out round pieces, place a little jam or marmalade in the middle, close up the dough, forming the dough nuts, and cook them in boiling oil or vege-butter until brown and thoroughly done. Eat warm.

GINGER SPONGE CAKE (a nice Cake for Children who do not like Gingerbread)

3 breakfast cups of Allinson wholemeal flour, I breakfast cup of sugar, 3 eggs, 6oz of butter or vege-butter, 2 heaped teaspoonfuls of ground ginger, I saltspoonful of salt, 1/2 gill milk.

Beat the butter, sugar, and eggs to a cream, mix all the dry ingredients together; add gradually to the butter, &c., lastly the milk. Put into a well-greased tin, bake for about 20 minutes in a quick oven. When cold cut into finger lengths or squares.

ICING FOR CAKES

To 8oz of sugar take 2 whites of eggs, well beaten, and I tablespoonful of orange-or rosewater.

Whisk the ingredients thoroughly, and when the cake is cold cover it with the mixture. Set the cake in the oven to harden, but do not let it remain long enough to discolour.

SEED CAKE

1/2lb fine wholemeal flour, 6oz butter, 6oz castor sugar, 2 eggs, 1/2oz carraway seeds.

Beat the butter and sugar to a cream, add the eggs well beaten, and dredge in the flour, add a little cold water it too dry. Bake for 1/2 an hour.

SPONGE CAKE ROLY-POLY

3 eggs, the weight of 2in fine wheatmeal, of 8in castor sugar, some raspberry and currant jam.

Beat up the eggs, sift in the sugar, then the flour. Line a large, square, flat baking tin with buttered paper, pour the mixture into it, and bake it in a fairly hot oven from 7 to 12 minutes, or until baked through. Have a sheet of white kitchen paper on the kitchen table, on which sprinkle some white sugar. Turn the cake out of the tin on to the paper, spread the cake with jam, and roll up. This should be done quickly, for if the cake is allowed to cool it will not roll.

UNFERMENTED FINGER-ROLLS

These are bread in the simplest and purest form, and liked by most. 1lb of Allinson wholemeal, a good $1/2$ pint of milk and water mixed.

Mix the meal and the milk and water into a dough, knead it a few minutes, then make the dough into finger-rolls on a floured pastry-board, rolling the finger-rolls about 3 inches long with the flat hand. Place them on a floured baking-tin, and bake them in a sharp oven from $1/2$ an hour to 1 hour. The time will depend on the heat of the oven. In a very hot oven the rolls will be well baked in $1/2$ an hour.

WHOLEMEAL BREAD (FERMENTED)

This will be found useful where a large family has to be provided for, or where it is desirable to bake bread for several days.

7lbs of Allinson wholemeal, $2^1/2$ pints of warm water (about 85° Faht.), 1 teaspoonful salt, $1/2$oz of yeast.

Dissolve the yeast in the water, add the salt, put the meal into a pan, make a hole in the centre of the meal, pour in the water with the yeast and salt, and mix the whole into a dough. Allow it to stand, covered with a cloth, 1 1/2 hours in front of the fire, turning the pan sometimes, so that the dough may get warm evenly. Then knead the dough well through, and if necessary add a little more warm water. Make the dough into round loaves, or fill it into greased tins, and bake it for 1 1/2 hours. The oven should be fairly hot. To know whether the bread is done, a clean skewer or knife should be passed through a loaf. If it comes out clean the bread is done; if it sticks it not sufficiently baked. When it is desired to have a soft crust, the loaves may be baked under tins in the oven.

WHOLEMEAL CAKE

1lb of wholemeal, 4oz of sugar, 1 teaspoonful of cinnamon, 1 breakfastcupful of currants and sultanas mixed, well-washed and picked over, 3oz of chopped sweet almonds, 1 dozen ground bitter almonds, 3 eggs, 1/2oz of German yeast, 1/2lb vege-butter, and some warm milk.

Rub the butter into the meal, add the fruit, cinnamon, almonds and sugar, and the eggs well beaten. Dissolve the yeast in a cupful of warm milk (not hot milk) add it to the other ingredients, and make all into a moist dough, adding as much more milk as is required to make the dough sufficiently moist for the spoon to beat all together. Cover the pan in which you mix the cake with a cloth, place it in front of the fire, and allow the dough to rise for 1 1/2 hours, turning the pan round occasionally that the dough may be equally warm. Then fill the dough into one or several well-greased tins, and bake the cake or cakes from 1 to 1 1/2 hours (according to the size) in a hot oven. If the cake browns too soon, cover it over with a sheet of paper.

Chapter 10

MENUS

VEGETARIANISM and hygienic living were a family business for the Allinsons. And it was Anna Allinson who devised menus for entertaining, a few of which are included here, prefaced by her own thoughts.

I have written the following menus to help those who are beginning vegetarianism. When first starting, most housewives do not know what to provide, and this is a source of anxiety. I occasionally meet some who have been vegetarians a long time, but confess that they do not know how to provide a nice meal. They usually eat the plainest foods, because they know of no tasty dishes. When visitors come, we like to provide tempting dishes for them, and show them that appetising meals can be prepared without the carcases of animals.

I have allowed three courses at the dinner, but they are really not necessary. I give them to make the menus more complete. A substantial soup and a pudding, or a savoury with vegetables and sauce and a pudding, are sufficient for a good meal. In our own household we rarely have more than two courses, and often only one course. This article will be of assistance to all those who are wishing to try a healthful and humane diet, and to those meat eaters who wish to provide tasty meals for vegetarian friends.

MENU 1

TOMATO SOUP

1 tin of tomatoes or 2lbs of fresh ones, 1 large Spanish onion or $^1/_2$lb of smaller ones, 2oz of butter, pepper and salt to taste, 1oz of vermicelli and 2 bay leaves.

Peel the onions and chop up roughly; brown them with the butter in the saucepan in which the soup is made. When the onion is browned, add the tomatoes (the fresh ones must be sliced) and 3 pints of water. Let all cook together for $^1/_2$ an hour. Then drain the liquid through a sieve without rubbing anything through. Return the liquid to the saucepan, add the seasoning and the vermicelli; then allow the soup to cook until the vermicelli is soft, which will be in about 10 minutes. Sago, tapioca, or a little dried julienne may be used instead of the vermicelli.

VEGETABLE PIE

$^1/_2$lb each of tomatoes, turnips, carrots, potatoes, 1 tablespoonful of sago, 1 teaspoonful of mixed herbs, 3 hard-boiled eggs, 2oz of butter, and pepper and salt to taste.

Prepare the vegetables, scald and skin the tomatoes, cut them in pieces not bigger than a walnut, stew them in the butter and 1 pint of water until nearly tender, add the pepper and salt and the mixed herbs. When cooked, pour the vegetables into a pie-dish, sprinkle in the sago, add water to make gravy if necessary. Cut the hard-boiled eggs in quarters and place them on the top of the vegetables, cover with a crust made from Allinson wholemeal, and bake until it is brown.

SHORT CRUST

10oz of Allinson wholemeal, 8oz of butter or vege-butter, 1 teacupful of cold water.

Rub the butter into the meal, add the water, mixing the paste with a knife. Roll it out, cut strips to line the rim of the pie-dish, cover the vegetable with the crust, decorate it, and bake the pie as directed.

GOLDEN SYRUP PUDDING

10oz of Allinson wholemeal, 3 eggs, 1 pint of milk, and $1/2$lb of golden syrup.

Grease a pudding basin, and pour the golden syrup into it; make a batter with the milk, meal, and eggs, and pour this into the pudding basin on the syrup, but do not stir the batter up with the syrup. Place a piece of buttered paper on the top of the batter, tie a cloth over the basin unless you have a basin with a fitting metal lid, and steam the pudding for $2^1/2$ hours in boiling water. Do not allow any water to boil into the pudding. Dip the basin with the pudding in it for 1 minute in cold water before turning it out, for then it comes out more easily.

MENU II

CLEAR CELERY SOUP

1 large head of celery or 2 small ones, 1 large Spanish onion, 2oz of butter, pepper and salt to taste, and 1 blade of mace.

Chop the onion and fry it brown in the butter (or vege-butter) in the saucepan in which the soup is to be made. When brown, add 4 pints of water, the celery washed and cut into pieces, the mace, the pepper and salt. Let all cook until the celery is quite soft, then drain the liquid from the vegetables. Return it to the saucepan, boil the soup up, and add 1oz of vermicelli, sago, or Italian paste; let the soup cook until this is quite soft, and serve with sippets of Allinson wholemeal toast.

BUTTER BEANS WITH PARSLEY SAUCE

Pick the beans, wash them and steep them over night in boiling water, just covering them. Allow 2 or 3oz of beans for each person. In the morning let them cook gently in the water they are steeped in, with the addition of a little butter, until quite soft, which will be in about 2 hours. The beans should be cooked in only enough water to keep them from burning; therefore, when it boils away, add only just sufficient for absorption. The sauce is made thus: I pint of milk, I tablespoonful of Allinson wholemeal, a handful of finely chopped parsley, the juice of 1/2 lemon, pepper and salt to taste. Boil the milk and thicken it with the meal, which should first be smoothed with a little cold milk, then last of all add the lemon juice, the seasoning, and the parsley. This dish should be eaten with potatoes and green vegetables.

GROUND RICE PUDDING

I quart of milk, 6oz of ground rice, I egg, and any kind of jam.

Boil the milk, stir into it the ground rice previously smoothed with some of the cold milk. Let the mixture cook gently for 5 minutes, stir frequently, draw the saucepan to the side, and when it has ceased to boil add the egg well whipped, and mix well. Pour half of the mixture into a pie-dish, spread a layer of jam over it, then pour the rest of the pudding mixture over the jam, and let it brown lightly in the oven.

MENU III

CARROT SOUP

4 good-sized carrots, I small head of celery, I fair sized onion, aturnip, 3oz of Allinson breadcrumbs, I 1/2oz of butter, I blade of mace, pepper and salt to taste. Scrape and wash the vegetables, and cut them up small; set them over the fire with 3 pints of water, the butter, bread, and

mace. Let all boil together until the vegetables are quite tender, and then rub them through a sieve. Return the mixture to the saucepan, season with pepper and salt, and if too thick add water to the soup, which should be as thick as cream. Boil the soup up, and serve.

CURRIED RICE AND TOMATOES

1/2lb of Patna rice, I dessertspoonful of curry powder, salt to taste, and Ioz of butter.

Wash the rice, put it over the fire in cold water, let it just boil up, then drain the water off. Mix I pint of cold water with the curry powder, put this over the fire with the rice, butter, and salt. Cover the rice with a piece of buttered paper and let it simmer gently until the water is absorbed. This will take about 20 minutes. Rice cooked this way will have all the grains separate. For the tomatoes proceed as follows: Ilb of tomatoes and a little butter, pepper, and salt. Wash the tomatoes and place them in a flat tin with a few spoonfuls of water; dust them with pepper and salt, and place little bits of butter on each tomato. Bake them from I5 to 20 minutes, according to the size of the tomatoes and the heat of the oven. Place the rice in the centre of a hot flat dish, put the tomatoes round it, pour the liquid over the rice, and serve.

APPLE CHARLOTTE

2lbs of cooking apples, I teacupful of mixed currants and sultanas, I heaped-up teaspoonful of ground cinnamon, 2oz of blanched and chopped almonds, sugar to taste, Allinson wholemeal bread, and butter.

Pare, core, and cut up the apples and set them to cook with a teacupful of water. Some apples require much more water than others. When they are soft add the fruit picked and washed, the cinnamon, and the almonds and sugar. Cut very thin slices of bread and butter, line a buttered pie-dish with them. Place a layer of apples over the buttered bread, and repeat the layers of bread and apples until the dish is full, finishing with a layer of bread and butter. Bake from $1/2$ of an hour to 1 hour.

WHOLESOME COOKERY

BREAKFASTS

As breakfast is the first meal of the day, it must vary in quantity and quality according to the work afterwards to be done. The literary man will best be suited with a light meal, whilst those engaged in hard work will require a heavier one. The clerk, student, businessman, or professional man, will find one of the three following breakfasts to suit him well:

I. Allinson wholemeal bread, 6 to 8oz, cut thick, with a scrape of butter; with this take from 6 to 8oz of ripe, raw fruit, or seasonable green stuff; at the end of the meal have a cup of cool, thin, and not too sweet cocoa, or Brunak*, or a cup of cool milk and water, bran tea, or even a cup of water that has been boiled and allowed to go nearly cold. An egg may be taken at this meal by those luxuriously inclined, and if not of a costive habit. The fruits allowed are all the seasonable ones, or dried prunes if there is a tendency to constipation. The green stuffs include watercress, tomatoes, celery, cucumber, and salads. Lettuce must be eaten sparingly at this meal, as it causes a sleepy feeling. Sugar must be used in strict moderation; jam, or fruits stewed with much sugar must be avoided, as they cause mental confusion and disinclination for brain work.

II. 3 to 4oz of Allinson wholemeal or crushed wheat, coarse oatmeal or groats, hominy, maize or barley meal may be boiled for $1/2$ an hour with milk and water, a very little salt being taken by those who use it. When ready, the porridge should be poured upon platters or soup-plates, allowed to cool, and then eaten with bread. Stewed fruits may be eaten with the porridge, or fresh fruit may be taken afterwards. When porridge is made with water, and then eaten with milk, too

* Brunak was a proprietary brand, no longer in existence.

much fluid enters the stomach, digestion is delayed, and waterbrash frequently occurs. Meals absorb at least thrice their weight of water in cooking, so that 4oz of meal will make at least 16oz of porridge. Sugar, syrup, treacle, or molasses should not be eaten with porridge, as they are apt to cause acid risings in the mouth, heartburn, and flatulence. In summer, wholemeal and barleymeal make the best porridges, and they may be taken cold; in autumn, winter, and early spring, oatmeal or hominy are the best, and may be eaten lukewarm. When porridges are eaten, no other course should be taken afterwards, but the entire meal should be made of porridge, bread, and fruit. Neither cocoa nor any other fluids should be taken after a porridge meal, or the stomach becomes filled with too much liquid, and indigestion results. To make the best-flavoured porridge, the coarse meal or crushed grain should be stewed in the oven for an hour or two; it may be made the day before it is required, and just warmed through before being brought to the table. This may be eaten with Allinson wholemeal bread and a small quantity of milk, or fresh or stewed fruit.

III. Cut 4 to 6oz of Allinson wholemeal bread into dice, put into a basin, and pour over about 1/2 a pint of boiling milk, or milk and water; cover the basin with a plate, let it stand ten minutes, and then eat slowly. Sugar or salt should not be added to the bread and milk. An apple, pear, orange, grapes, banana, or other seasonable fruit may be eaten afterwards. No other foods should be eaten at this meal, but only the bread, milk, and fruit.

Labourers, artisans, and those engaged in hard physical work may take any of the above breakfasts. If they take No. I, they may allow themselves from 8 to 10oz of bread, and should drink a large cup of Brunak afterwards, as their work requires a fair amount of liquid to carry off some of the heat caused by the burning up of food whilst they are at work. If No. II breakfast is taken, 6 to 8oz of meal may be allowed. If No. III breakfast is eaten, then 6 or 8oz of bread and 2 pint of milk may be taken.

N.B.–Women require about a quarter less food than men do, and must arrange the quantity accordingly.

MIDDAY MEALS

The meal in the middle of the day must vary according to the work to be done after it. If much mental strain has to be borne or business done, the meal must be a light one, and should be lunch rather than dinner. Those engaged in hard physical work should make their chief meal about midday, and have a light repast in the evening.

LUNCH: One of the simplest lunches is that composed of Allinson wholemeal bread and fruit. From 6 to 8oz of bread may be eaten, and about $1/2$lb of any raw fruit that is in season; afterwards a glass of lemon water or bran tea, Brunak, or a cup of thin, cool, and not too sweet cocoa may be taken, or a tumbler of milk and water slowly sipped. The fruit may be advantageously replaced by a salad, which is a pleasant change from fruit, and sits as lightly on the stomach. Wholemeal biscuits and fruit, with a cup of fluid, form another good lunch. A basin of any kind of porridge with milk, but without sugar, also makes a light and good midday repast; or a basin of thin vegetable soup and bread, or macaroni, or even plain vegetables. The best lunch of all will be found in Allinson wholemeal bread, and salad or fruit, as it is not wise to burden the system with too much cooked food, and one never feels so light after made dishes as after bread and fruit.

Labouring men who wish to take something with them to work will find 12oz of Allinson wholemeal bread, $1/2$lb fresh fruit, and a large mug of Brunak or cocoa satisfy them well; or instead of cocoa they may have milk and water, lemon water, lemonade, oatmeal water, or some harmless non-alcoholic drink. Another good meal is made from $1/2$lb of the wholemeal bread and butter, and a $1/2$lb of peas pudding spread between the slices. The peas can be flavoured with a little pepper, salt, and mustard by those who still cling to condiments. 12oz of the wholemeal bread, 2 or 3oz of cheese, some raw fruit, or an onion, celery, watercress, or other greenstuff, with a large cup of fluid, form another good meal. $1/2$lb of coarse oatmeal or crushed wheat made into porridge the day before, and warmed up at midday, will last a man well until he gets home at night. Or a boiled bread pudding may be taken to work, warmed and eaten. This is made from the wholemeal bread, which is soaked in hot water until soft, then crushed or crumbled, some currants or raisins are then mixed with this, a little soaked sago stirred in; lastly, a very little sugar and spice are added as a flavouring. This mixture is then tied up in a pudding cloth and boiled, or it may be put in a pudding basin covered with a cloth, and boiled in a saucepan. A pleasing addition to this pudding is some finely chopped almonds, or Brazil nuts.

DINNERS

As dinner is the chief meal of the day it should consist of substantial food. It may be taken in the middle of the day by those who work hard; but if taken at night, at least five hours must elapse before going to bed, so that the stomach may have done its work before sleep comes on.

A dinner may consist of many courses or different dishes, but the simpler the dishes and the less numerous the courses the better. A person who makes his meal from one dish only is the wisest of all. He who limits himself to two courses does well, but he who takes more than three courses lays up for himself stomach troubles or disorder of the system. When only one course is had, then good solid food must be eaten; when two courses are the rule, a moderate amount of each should be taken; and if three different dishes are provided, a proportionately lighter quantity of each. Various dishes may be served for the dinner meal, such as soups, omelettes, savouries, pies, batters, and sweet courses.

The plainest dinner any one can eat is that composed of Allinson wholemeal bread and raw fruit. A man in full work may eat from 12 to 16oz of the wholemeal bread, and about the same quantity of ripe raw fruit. The bread is best dry, the next best is when a thin scrape of butter is spread on it. If hard physical work has to be done, a cup of Brunak, cocoa, milk and water, or lemon water, should be drunk at the end of the meal. In winter these fluids might be taken warmed, but in summer they are best cool or cold. This wholesome fare can be varied in a variety of ways; some might like a salad instead of the fruit, and others may prefer cold vegetables. A few Brazil nuts, almonds, walnuts, some Spanish nuts, or a piece of cocoanut may be eaten with the bread in winter. Others not subject to piles, constipation, or eczema, &c, may take 2oz of cheese and an onion with their bread, or a hard-boiled egg. This simple meal can be easily carried to work, or on a journey. Wholemeal biscuits or Allinson rusks may be used instead of bread if one is on a walking tour, cycling trip, or boating excursion, or even on ordinary occasions for a change.

Of cooked dinners, the simplest is that composed of potatoes baked, steamed, or boiled in their skins, eaten with another vegetable, sauce, and the wholemeal bread. Baked potatoes are the most wholesome, and their skins should always be eaten; steamed potatoes are next; whilst boiled ones, especially if peeled, are not nearly so good. Any seasonable vegetable may be steamed and eaten with the potatoes, such as cauliflower, cabbage, sprouts, broccoli, carrot, turnip, beetroot, parsnips, or boiled celery, or onions. Recipes for the sauces used with this course will be found in another part of the book; they may be parsley, onion, caper, tomato, or brown gravy sauce. This dinner may be varied by adding to it a poached, fried, or boiled egg. As a second course, baked apples, or stewed fresh fruit and bread may be eaten; or Allinson bread pudding, or rice, sago, tapioca, or macaroni pudding with stewed fruit. Persons troubled with piles, varicose veins, varicocele, or constipation must avoid this dinner as much as possible. If they do eat it they must be sure to eat the skins of the potatoes, and take the Allinson bread pudding or bread and fruit afterwards, avoiding puddings of rice, sago, tapioca, or macaroni.

EVENING MEAL
Evening meal or tea meal should be the last meal at which solid food is eaten. It should always be a light one, and the later it is eaten the less substantial it should be. Heavy or hard work after tea is no excuse for a supper. This meal must be taken at least three hours before retiring. From 4 to 6oz of Allinson wholemeal bread may be allowed with a poached or lightly boiled egg, a salad, or fruit, or some kind of green food. The fluid drunk may be Brunak, cocoa, milk and water, bran tea, or even plain water, boiled and taken cool. Those who are restless at night, nervous, or sleepless must not drink tea at this meal. Fruit in the

evening is not considered good, and when taken it should be cooked rather than raw. Boiled celery will be found to be lighter on the stomach at this meal than the raw vegetable. When it is boiled, as little water as possible should be used; the water that the celery is boiled in may be thickened with Allinson fine wheatmeal, made into sauce, and poured over the cooked celery; by this means we do not loose the valuable salts dissolved out of the food by boiling. Mustard and cress, watercress, radishes, and spring onions may be eaten if the evening meal is taken 4 or 5 hours before going to bed. Those who are away from home all day, and who take their food to their work may have some kind of milk pudding at this meal. Wheatmeal blancmange, or cold milk pudding may occasionally be eaten. Those who are costive will find a boiled onion or some braized onions very useful. Boil the onion in as little water as possible and serve up with the liquor it is boiled in. To prepare braized onions, fry them first until nicely brown, using butter or olive oil, then add a cupful of boiling water to the contents of the frying pan, cover with a plate, and let cook for an hour. This is not really a rich food, but one easy of digestion and of great use to the sleepless. Those who want to rise early must make their last meal a light one. Those troubled with dreams or restlessness must do the same. Very little fluid should be taken last thing at night, as it causes persons to rise frequently to empty the bladder.

SUPPERS
Hygienic livers will never take such meals, even if tea has been early, or hard work done since the tea meal was taken. No solid food must be eaten. The most that should be consumed is a cup of Brunak, cocoa, lemon water, bran tea, or even boiled water, but never milk. In winter warm drinks may be taken, and in summer cool ones.

DRINKS
LEMON WATER: is made by squeezing the juice of $1/2$ a lemon into a tumbler of warm or cold water; to this is added just enough sugar to take off the tartness. Some peel the lemon first, then cut in slices, pour boiling water over the slices, grate in a little of the peel, and add sugar to taste.

BRUNAK: Take 1 1/2 to 2 teaspoonfuls of Brunak for each large cupful required, mix it with sufficient water, and boil for 2 or 3 minutes to get the full flavour, then strain and add hot milk and sugar to taste. Can be made in a coffee-pot, teapot, or jug if preferred. May be stood on the hob to draw; or it you have any left over from a previous meal it can be boiled up again and served as freshly made.

COCOA: This is best made by putting a teaspoonful of any good cocoa, such as Allinson's, into a breakfast cup; boiling water is then poured upon this and stirred; 1 tablespoonful of milk must be added to each cup, and 1 teaspoonful of sugar where sugar is used, or 1 or 2 teaspoonfuls of condensed milk and no extra sugar.

BRAN TEA: Mix 1oz of bran with 1 pint of water; boil for 1/2 an hour, strain, and drink cool. A little orange or lemon juice is a pleasant addition. When this is used as a drink at breakfast or tea, a little milk and sugar may be added to it.

CHOCOLATE: Allow 1 bar of Allinson's chocolate for each cup of fluid. Break the chocolate in bits, put into a saucepan, add a little boiling water, put on the fire, and stir until the chocolate is dissolved, then add rest of fluid and boil 2 or 3 minutes. Pour the chocolate into cups, and add about 1 tablespoonful of fresh milk to each cup, but no extra sugar. The milk may be added to the chocolate whilst boiling, if desired.

RECIPE INDEX

INDEX